Start Here

7 Easy, Diet-Free Steps to Achieving Your Ultimate Health and Happiness

Megan Lyons

BY MEGAN LYONS

THANK YOU!

As a thank you for purchasing this book, please visit **www.StartHereBonus.com** for four exclusive, 100 percent FREE bonus gifts. You will find:

- The *Lyons' Share Healthy Pantry Guide* to fill your cabinets with the items that will set you up for health success.

- The *"Start Here, Star There" Health Tracker* to ensure you stay motivated and consistent with the practices you'll learn about in this book.

- Entry to an encouraging and supportive accountability group on Facebook, only for readers of *Start Here*.

- The *Lyons' Share Weekly Meal Planner* template to quickly and easily plan your week of healthy meals.

COPYRIGHT

Start Here: 7 Easy, Diet-Free Steps to Achieving Your Ultimate Health and Happiness

Disclaimer:

This book is not intended as a substitute for medical advice. The reader should regularly consult a physician in matters relating to his/her health, and particularly with respect to any symptoms that may require diagnosis or medical attention. The exercises and advice in this book are given for informational purposes only. Consult a physician before performing this or any exercise program.

The content of this book is for general instruction only. Each person's physical, emotional, and spiritual condition is unique. The instruction in this book is not intended to replace or interrupt the reader's relationship with a physician or other professional. Please consult your doctor for matters pertaining to your specific health and diet.

To contact the author, visit http://www.thelyonsshare.org or email Megan@ TheLyonsShare.org.

ISBN: 978-0-9861332-0-6

Printed in the United States of America

CONTENTS

"Every journey begins with a single step"

— Maya Angelou

ACKNOWLEDGMENTS

I've heard it said that the first book is the hardest, and Roald Dahl even said, "a person is a fool to become a writer." Developing the ideas, tips, and advice in this book wasn't difficult at all (I have dozens and dozens of books' worth of ideas to share!), but the process of actually making the book a reality was challenging. With a thriving client practice, a constant influx of emails awaiting responses, and an incessant desire to fill my schedule to the brim, setting aside time to write (and then sticking to it) didn't happen as quickly as I'd have liked. Still, the fact that you are reading this now means that I've done it, and I'm so thrilled to be sharing my thoughts, tips, and motivation with you through these pages. Thank you for reading!

There are several people to thank for their help in creating or inspiring this book:

First, of course, to my husband, Kevin, who didn't bat an eye when I said I wanted to leave my well-paying job to start the business of my dreams, and has supported me every single day since. He not only sits through my business reviews and listens to my lofty goals and dreams, but also lives through the dramatic highs and lows that every entrepreneur feels, and believes that I will succeed just as much as I do. For the hours that I spent writing this book when I should have been spending time with you, and for being my unwavering rock and best supporter, Kev, I thank you so much.

Thank you also to the rest of my family, who constantly encourage and support me. My Mom and Dad still think I hung the moon in the sky, and would be by my side in anything I chose to do. My sister, Lindsey, and I have to constantly remind each other not to work so hard (I guess we do share the same genes!), and she may never know how much she inspired my own health journey through her own journey and her reaction to my first attempt at health. It is a huge understatement to say I won the in-law lottery in picking up Pat, Gary, Holly, and Teddy, and I appreciate your support, personally and professionally. You are the first to "like" my posts on Facebook, comment on my blog, participate in my programs, and ask how the business is going. Katie, Brian, Scott, and Jenni, thank you for being the supportive siblings you are, and especially for letting the best nephew and nieces in the world be a part of my life!

Thank you to the Institute for Integrative Nutrition Book Course, which got the writing process started, and Hal Elrod's Best Month Ever Challenge, which inspired me to pick up writing after a seven month break and actually finish the book.

Finally, thank you to my clients, who I am so lucky to serve. You have been the lab rats for many of the ideas in this book, and your success inspires me every single day to keep doing what I'm doing. I truly love being able to be a part of your lives, and I thank you for sharing them with me.

Start Here

7 Easy, Diet-Free Steps to Achieving Your Ultimate Health and Happiness

Chapter One

You Are Not Alone

f you feel stressed about your health nearly every day, ***you're not alone***. If you've tried to start "getting healthy" over and over again, made multiple New Year's resolutions that haven't quite stuck, or ridden the "diet roller coaster" up and down and back up again more times than you can count ... ***you're not alone***. If you know you want to start living a healthier lifestyle, but haven't been able to actually commit to changing, ***you're not alone***. If you are overwhelmed by so much conflicting information in the popular press and confused when health experts contradict each other nearly every minute ... ***you are not alone!***

Health is a problem that we all think about. In fact, the International Food Information Council Foundation's *2014 Food & Health Survey* reported that 91 percent of people have given "a little or a lot of thought" to the healthfulness of their foods and beverages over the past year.[1] Everywhere we turn, someone is talking about the latest diet fad, and diet commercials pop up almost as frequently as prescription drug commercials. Alluring headlines are splashed across grocery store tabloids everywhere. We've all seen that magazine promising: "Lose 20 pounds in a day by eating whatever you want!" and at least wondered if such a thing were actually possible. We are constantly inundated by messages telling us that if we don't look like a supermodel, we're not good enough.

Thinking so much about health goals that seem unreachable often causes feelings of guilt, stress, and anxiety. Many Americans live with constant health goals, go through a rotating cycle of fad diets, and always have "something we're working on" related to our health. Fifty-four percent of respondents in the *Food & Health Survey* said they were actively trying to lose weight right at the moment.

We Have a Problem

Truthfully, we have a problem as a society. Globally, the incidence of obesity has nearly doubled since 1980.[2] About two-thirds of adults in the U.S. are overweight or obese.[3] Sixty-five percent of the world's population currently lives in an area where being overweight or obese kills more people than being underweight. More than 100 million Americans are diabetic or pre-diabetic, and diabetes growth rates have tripled in the past 30 years.[4] The statistics go on and on, but suffice it to say that what we are doing isn't working.

In fact, no country has succeeded in decreasing obesity in the past 33 years.[5] Not one! Let that sink in, and then think about why we haven't been able to reverse our ever-expanding waistlines.

First, health is confusing. Or, at least, it's made to seem confusing by the popular press. There is always a new study showing that a food we formerly considered "healthy" is now linked to high cholesterol or contributes to obesity. There is always a new diet plan showing amazing results by eating a specific combination of foods, or a new pill promising to help you shed weight without changing anything about your diet or lifestyle. This sensationalism can make it seem impossible to figure out what is actually healthy. In fact, in 2012, half of those polled believed it was easier to do their taxes than to figure out how to eat healthfully.[6]

Second, we have been so focused on finding a "miracle diet" that we have lost sight of what actually nourishes our bodies. Think about the diet trends you have heard about in the past several decades. The 1990s featured several variations of low-fat diets. Ostensibly, we could eat as many fat-free (but sugar-laden) Snackwell's cookies as we wanted and still lose weight, as long as we avoided fat. Fat-free baked goods, fat-free meals, fat-free dairy, fat-free dressings, and more lined our pantries, yet we still had a weight problem. In fact, the weight problem got dramatically worse during the low-fat craze, leaving Americans searching for the next "miracle" solution.

We quickly rebounded by making carbohydrates out to be "evil." Popularized by Dr. Atkins, but mimicked by many similar diets, the low-carb craze encouraged Americans to eat all the bacon and cheese they desired, but to limit carbohydrates at any cost – meaning that, in the strictest phases, even vegetables and fruits were to be avoided. Guess what? A vast majority of those who succeeded in losing weight on low-carb diets gained even more back after they returned to normal eating patterns. And yes, we still had a weight problem.

Since that time, we have cycled through the South Beach Diet, the Zone Diet, Weight Watchers, the Paleo diet, the No White diet, the gluten-free diet, and hundreds more. We've been told we can eat as much as we want and not exercise if we take some miracle pills, and we've been told that eating processed, gluten-free versions of our favorite treats would solve our problems once and for all. Yet, we still have a weight problem.

We Need a Solution that Works, Not Another Fad Diet

Why are none of these working? First, so many of these diets forget that our bodies actually need real nutrition to function optimally. We need fat, we need protein, and, yes, we even need carbohydrates (although we are much better suited to getting our carbohydrates primarily from fruits and vegetables, rather than candy and unending pasta bowls). So many of the previously mentioned diets forget about balance, and instead focus on what to eliminate. Their alluring promises make us forget about real nutrition.

We can trick our bodies into losing weight in the short term by eliminating a food group or changing up our routine. For example, if we restrict intake of dietary fat, our body will try to utilize the fat stored on our bodies to take care of critical body processes. This will help us lose weight in the short term. In the long term, though, our organs will start to function less than optimally, our skin will become ashen, our hair will lose its natural shine, and our energy levels will plummet. And even if we lose weight initially, we'll end up gaining that weight back, or we'll end up with the look commonly known as "skinny fat," which basically involves a smaller frame but a flabbier, less toned build. Surely an untoned body and tanking energy levels cannot be our goal!

The second reason that fad diets don't work is that they often rely heavily on packaged and processed foods. It makes sense (financial sense, at least) that a company like Weight Watchers would have to produce products to make money. The products they produce fit into the calorie limits they have set up, but by any other standards cannot be considered "real food." The abundance of chemicals, preservatives, and machine-generated "food" in these products confuses our bodies. We are simply not able to utilize the nutrients from foods with ingredient lists a mile long as easily as we can use the nutrients from an apple or an almond. In the absence of nutrients it recognizes, the body can continue to crave more and more food, hoping to be given real nutrition. In the end, though, we often end up storing the excess energy as fat. To be honest, I think Weight Watchers is the lesser of many evils on the market – I'm not intending to pick on them, only to use a popular example.

The final reason fad diets don't work is probably the most critical. We simply can't stay on a restrictive diet forever, and we always rebound from that restriction. Once we're "off" the diet, we go back to our normal ways of eating immediately. In fact, we may rebound by eating even worse, if the diet has made us feel deprived.

This cycle of indulge-restrict-indulge-restrict (and so on) leads us to the vicious diet roller coaster, and can lead to a host of long-term health complications. In fact, studies show that those who yo-yo diet regularly end up *gaining* more weight over time than those who never diet.[7] What's worse, yo-yo dieting can desensitize our bodies' ability to regulate our hunger, our blood sugar levels, and our cravings. Eventually, yo-yo dieting may even lead to the development of Type 2 diabetes and other serious conditions.[8]

It Doesn't Have to Be That Complicated

Wouldn't it be nice to not have to worry about losing weight? To know that you have a few healthy behaviors that are sustainable and not too overwhelming? To live every day feeling energized, knowing what foods make you feel good, and actually enjoying them?

You're in the right place to begin working toward all of these goals, without feeling overwhelmed by every scientific detail. Of course, there is a lot to learn about nutrition, and I find the changes and updates fascinating. But this is my *job*, and so I need to stay tuned into the ever-changing research. If you don't have energy, time, or desire to deal with all of that, you're in the right place.

I'm here to tell you that **it just doesn't have to be that complicated.** There are simple things you can do to improve your health dramatically, help you shed excess weight, and have consistently stable energy ... *without* worrying about what the latest magazine says.

Think about your grandmother's grandmother, and the many generations that came before her. These people likely didn't know what a refined carbohydrate was (mostly because processed foods didn't exist!). They didn't bog themselves down by worrying about whether the Atkins Diet or the Master Cleanse was the right choice for them. They simply ate – whole, real, unprocessed foods. And their body's hunger mechanisms were in-tune enough to regulate their appetites so that they stopped when their nutrient needs were met.

We can enjoy the same food freedom, but we'll have to get over a few hurdles. First, the abundance of processed, chemical-infused "food" out there makes it tempting to grab a quick-fix, a tasty looking product inconspicuously labeled "healthy," a variety of items proclaiming that they are "low-carb," "heart-healthy," or "diet-friendly." We all live busy lives – and sometimes it's easier to rely on those products rather than slicing up a cucumber for a snack or making a smoothie for breakfast. And second, our bodies have been so beaten up and confused by our never-ending cycles of fad dieting, restriction, cravings, and chemicalized food products that they don't always help us to self-regulate our intakes anymore.

We **can** get back there, though. All it takes is returning our focus to the basics, and sticking to the set of 7 principles that I'll lay out in this book. I feel confident that if you follow these 7 steps, you'll not only feel better, get closer to your ideal weight, and have more energy – but you'll also feel relieved that you don't have to deal with the ups and downs any more. It's time to get off that diet roller coaster, and focus on real, nutritious food!

My Story

This book is about you – about finding the health habits that will make you feel your healthiest and happiest. As such, I won't bore you with pages upon pages of my own personal story. But I want to share the basics, so you know that these practices came to me over time. I wasn't born eating this way, and I've been through my ups and downs just as you may have.

As I was growing up, I was fortunate to have a mother who cared more about my sister and me than anyone else in the world. She went to drastic lengths to ensure we were fed and happy, and tried to give us balanced, nutritious meals. The problem was that none of us actually knew that much about real nutrition. So, the fact that I had a foil-wrapped breakfast to chow down in the car on the way to 5:30 a.m. dance practice was far more important than what I was actually eating.

Due to my busy schedule, I probably ate more meals in the car than at the dinner table, which is an issue in itself. To make matters worse, my meals focused on refined carbohydrates and lacked the nutrients that I encourage families today to include. A standard day-in-the-life for me might have been a breakfast of a bowl of oatmeal or a cinnamon sugar frosted Pop-Tart with butter (yes, I'm serious), a lunch of a turkey sandwich with a bag of pretzels and a cookie, and a dinner of spaghetti and meat sauce or meatloaf, mashed potatoes, and broccoli.

Throughout middle school and high school, I danced a lot – sometimes up to 20 hours a week between ballet, tap, jazz, and drill team practice. So, I never had to worry about my weight, my energy levels were fairly high (despite a major lack of sleep), and I ate as I pleased.

Near the end of high school, though, my eating habits changed. Just as I stopped dancing and lived a more sedentary life, I started hanging out with people who drank alcohol and ate fast food, and I joined them. I began eating out at restaurants a lot more and relying on packaged foods to sustain me in between meals. My weight steadily climbed, and when I walked onto campus my freshman year of college, I had gained 15-20 pounds fairly quickly.

I was never overweight by most people's standards, but I did not feel great about myself. An extra 15-20 pounds on a 5' 5" frame is quite a bit of weight, and for the first time in my life, I found myself thinking about incorporating exercise for the sake of exercise, and trying to figure out what healthy food actually was.

Fate must have had a heavy hand in introducing me to my now-husband, Kevin, on move-in day at Harvard, just as I was feeling lethargic and puffy. Kevin was on the track and cross country teams at school, and his life revolved around running. He was fit and seemed healthy, so as we started dating, I decided to pick up running in hopes that it would make me healthy, too.

No sugar-coating here – I hated running. I stuck with it, since I really liked Kevin and wanted to impress him, but it wasn't fun. Even as I improved a bit in my endurance (going from a quarter-mile, slowly, to being able to run a mile without stopping), my body wasn't reacting the way I wanted it to. I was missing the biggest piece of the puzzle – nutrition.

I began "learning" about nutrition the way most people do – with popular magazines. They seemed to think that calorie restriction and hours on the elliptical machine were the key to happiness, so I went down that path for a while. Breaking off half of a processed protein bar for lunch and pedaling away on the elliptical for 90 minutes a day, I did end up losing weight.

Too much weight, in fact. My new "healthy" lifestyle became addicting, and I eventually found myself controlling every morsel of food I put into my body. I made decisions based on reducing calories rather than optimizing health, such as choosing a diet bar (loaded with artificial sweeteners, chemicals, and preservatives) over a healthy, balanced meal.

Not only was I obsessed with the idea of controlling my food, but my energy was also flagging terribly. I lost the "pep in my step" that I had always had, since my body did not have the nutrition it needed. Still, the cycle of restriction is tempting, and as I continued to see results, it was hard to break myself of the restrictive behavior.

I was fortunate to break free of my restrictive cycle with urging from Kevin and my family, as well as a genuine interest in what real nutrition was. By reading dozens of books on real nutrition, and immersing myself in studies of how our bodies actually utilized food, I eventually broke free of the restrictive cycle, and finally found my own healthy and happy weight.

For the 12 years since that time, I've learned more and more about nutrition, and my own diet has evolved considerably. I consider nutrition an ongoing study, and I love trying new things on myself, So I don't think I'll ever fall into a routine of eating that will stay with me for the rest of my life. I dislike labels for the sake of labels, and think people too easily fall into calling themselves "Paleo" or "vegan" just to sound healthy, without making decisions that are truly making their bodies feel the best. So, I don't have a label, and I like it that way. I eat meat (though I try to prioritize high-quality meat when possible, and I keep my portion sizes under control), I eat grains (though they are almost never the focus of my meal), I eat sugar (because, let's be realistic, life happens! But I still try to keep my intake under control, since I know the impact it has on my body). I eat at restaurants when I have occasions to do so (though

I honestly prefer cooking my own food). I don't panic when I have to travel and don't know what I'll be eating. I enjoy holidays to the fullest. My daily diet changes constantly according to my goals, my preferences, and what's going on in my life.

Still, I've absolutely never felt better. I weigh myself periodically – around every week – and my weight has stayed fairly consistent for the last 12 years. This is all *without* being on a diet, feeling restrictive, or denying myself things I truly want to eat.

Even better than the weight, I feel great. People often call me "The Energizer Bunny," or comment that I have more energy than they could possibly muster in a lifetime. This is just normal for me – I love living a busy and active life, which includes some form of exercise almost every day. I have found the nutrition balance that gives me energy to power through every day and feel my best.

The running that I hated at the beginning of college has become a passion. Running, to me, is a way to escape the stresses of day-to-day life, honor my need for "me time," be outside in nature, reflect, move my body, and enjoy. Because I always seek continuous improvement in my own life, my first 5K race turned into a 10K, which turned into a half marathon and then a marathon. Since I started running, I have completed 5 marathons, more than 30 half marathons, a Half Ironman duathlon, several triathlons, and dozens of smaller races. I'll never make the Olympics, and may never win a race, but the competition against myself is addictive, fun, and energizing.

My knowledge of real nutrition has grown significantly, as well. While getting my MBA at Northwestern's Kellogg School of Management, I enrolled at the Institute for Integrative Nutrition, which was the beginning of my true, unbridled passion for helping others get healthy. IIN taught me more than 100 dietary theories, with compelling research from every single one ... leading me to the conclusion that there is no one, single "perfect diet." IIN taught me self-compassion and self-love, and how intricately emotions are tied in with our diets. Most importantly, IIN taught me that I could help others achieve their ultimate health and happiness. (If you are interested in an education at IIN, please contact me at megan@ thelyonsshare.org. As an Ambassador, I frequently get significant discounts to give out to my followers.)

Once I graduated from IIN (and from Kellogg), I returned to my previous job of management consulting. I was good at the job, and enjoyed helping companies become more efficient and profitable. But something was missing. I continued to daydream about helping others achieve health, and continued to spend every waking moment enrolled in continuing education nutrition courses, reading nutrition books, and talking to friends and family about nutrition.

It is this passion that ultimately led me to start my own business, The Lyons' Share Wellness, where I now spend every day helping others achieve their ultimate health and happiness. My job is primarily composed of one-on-one health coaching, where I work with clients to find a nutrition and lifestyle balance that works for them. My clients' successes have been mind-blowing (see the "Testimonials" section and the "About The Lyons' Share Wellness" section at the end of this book), and working to guide people to their ultimate health and happiness is my true passion.

In the spirit of continuing to explore and learn, I am also in the process of completing my master's in Holistic Nutrition through Hawthorn University. I will always be hungry for more knowledge, and this advanced degree is exactly what I was craving. In my master's program, I am learning the intricate science behind the nutrition principles that I already have been incorporating into my clients' lessons, and rounding out my knowledge so that I can even better serve every unique client that walks through my doors.

The common ground through all of my experiences is that I love to help others achieve health. I have seen a lot – from a client whose diet consisted of only pork rinds and red wine to a client who frequently consumed several dozen candy bars in a stressful situation; from clients who were eating "perfect" diets, yet couldn't lose the belly fat, to a young client who was throwing up daily and had been dismissed by traditional doctors. I've learned a lot from all of these situations, and while they were all unique, there are several common threads that tie them all together. These common threads are the 7 principles that I lay out in this book, and I am completely confident that they will help you achieve a higher level of health and happiness – just as they helped me, and as they helped my clients.

You Don't Have to Eat Less, You Just Have to Eat Better

Throughout this book, I'll make several recommendations that will help you improve your nutrition. You'll see that the suggestions I make will not be complicated, and you may find yourself doubting that something so simple could actually succeed in improving your health. This is probably because the popular media has convinced you that losing weight is all about restricting your food intake as much as possible. So-called health magazines often will imply that it's good to be starving throughout the day, and that you should reward yourself for eating as little as possible in order to lose weight.

My approach is dramatically different. In fact, now that I know more about nutrition and consider my diet an overall healthy one, I probably eat *more* food than I ever ate before. It's not unusual for my dinner to require more than one plate, or for my lunch to require multiple Tupperware containers. I'm an active, busy person, and I exercise a lot, so I do need a lot of food. Plus, I really enjoy eating, and there's nothing wrong with that!

The difference is that the majority of my food today is very high-quality, nutrient-rich, whole food. By eating mostly vegetables, fruits, and other nutritious and naturally occurring foods, you can actually eat a lot *more* than you may have been led to believe!

Our bodies need calories for energy, but we also need nutrients for each of our cells to function optimally. When we feed ourselves processed foods that are usually devoid of any significant nutrition, our bodies still crave the antioxidants and phytonutrients that keep it running well, so it's harder and harder to feel full. The popular slogan "Once you pop, you just can't stop" rings sadly true, as you've probably realized if you've eaten an entire sleeve of chips or cookies, only to feel like you could easily go back for another.

When we feed ourselves nutrient-dense food, though, our hunger mechanisms are pretty good at telling us when to stop. After all, it's nearly impossible to eat 1,000 calories worth of cucumbers in a sitting (that would be over 22 whole cucumbers!), but eating 3.5 rich chocolate chip cookies doesn't seem out of the question.

I believe you should never deprive yourself of food if you are truly feeling hungry. Do not begin this book thinking that you should starve yourself when you are hungry, or eat less in order to lose weight. As long as you are eating the right foods, I truly believe you can lose weight and feel your best by eating even more quantity than you currently consume.

The Mystery of Bioindividuality

One of my very favorite principles from my education at the Institute for Integrative Nutrition is the concept of "bioindividuality." Simply put, bioindividuality means that there is no one perfect diet that suits every person on the planet, and one person's food may very well be another person's poison. Think about the dramatic differences in the diets of native Alaskan Eskimos (very high protein and fat, including lots of whale blubber and animal products, with very little fruit or grains, and relatively few vegetables) versus the highly touted diet of the Mediterranean culture (very high in fruits, vegetables, olive oil, beans, grains, and fish). Yet, both cultures boast some of the healthiest people on the planet.

One of the main reasons that so many of the fad diets we have discussed can produce scientific studies promising that their diet is "*the solution*" is that there isn't a single diet that works for everyone. Some might thrive on a high-protein diet, while others do better with a higher carbohydrate intake. Some feel great as vegans, while others feel unsatisfied if a meal doesn't contain an animal product.

Bioindividuality means that you need to experiment with exactly what combination of foods suits you best. It takes experimentation with a variety of different eating styles, and your ideal diet may change over time. Some people who have put themselves through several years of restriction, yo-yo dieting, or strict adherence to specific diet plans might find it hard to be sufficiently in-tune to their bodies to truly know what makes them feel best. For these people, seeking the advice of a health coach or other health professional may be the best course of action.

Although I believe wholeheartedly in bioindividuality, the concept makes it impossible to write a book that would prescribe the perfect diet for each one of my readers. For this reason, I have boiled down my knowledge of nutrition into the 7 concepts that I am confident will work for an overwhelming majority of people. I have yet to find a health-coaching client who has not seen dramatic results (in terms of weight loss, increased energy, improved digestion, reduction of fatigue, or a wide variety of other symptoms) by implementing these 7 tips. I feel completely confident in recommending these 7 tips to you, despite knowing that your ideal diet may be very different than that of another person reading this book.

The Seven Steps

Wouldn't it be nice to not have to worry about losing weight? To know that you have a few healthy behaviors that are sustainable and not too overwhelming? To live every day feeling energized, knowing what foods make you feel good, and actually enjoying them?

You're in the right place to get started working toward all of the goals. Through the course of this book, I will share seven steps to improve your health easily, and in a sustainable way. If you follow each of these seven steps, I am confident that you'll feel better physically, and also feel inspired to continue your health journey. These are the first seven steps to achieving your ultimate health and happiness!

The seven steps we will discuss are:

1. Hydrate adequately

2. Increase consumption of vegetables

3. Reduce added sugar

4. Make it work for your situation

5. Make exercise a priority

6. Practice gratitude and self-forgiveness

7. Seek accountability

A chapter on each of the seven steps follows this chapter.

Prepare for Positive Change

We are about to cover a lot of health and nutrition information. I hope that you'll learn a lot, be inspired to make positive changes for your own health, and jump-start your own continual improvement as a result of what you learn here.

What I hope you do *not* do as a result of the upcoming chapters is beat yourself up about your previous habits. Remember, comparison is the thief of joy, and there is value in appreciating where you are today. So, when I tell you in Chapter Two how much water you should drink for optimal health, don't think about what a poor job of hydration you've done up until this point. Instead, think about the potential benefits of drinking water, and how great you'll feel when you start implementing this change.

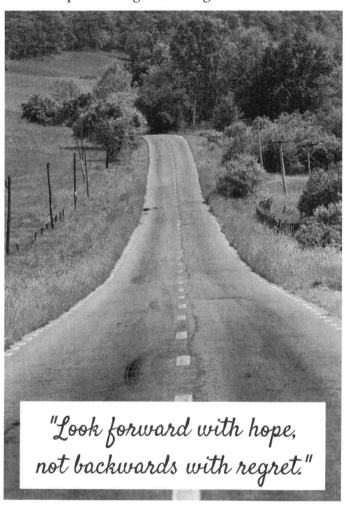

"*Look forward with hope, not backwards with regret.*"

So sit back, relax, and prepare to make changes to your health that will make you feel your healthiest and happiest. I hope you finish this book feeling motivated to take your health into your own hands, inspired that the right path for you just doesn't have to be as complicated as the popular media might make it seem, and excited to implement changes in your own diet. Most of all, I hope you finish this book realizing that you are capable of feeling great and being in control of your health and nutrition. If you approach this with an open mind and follow these 7 simple steps, I know you will feel more energized, healthy, and vibrant!

To make the most of your journey through *Start Here*, I recommend joining our supportive and encouraging community at **www. StartHereCommunity.com**. You'll find others at similar stages in their journeys, and be able to encourage and motivate each other to achieve your goals!

CHAPTER TWO

QUENCH YOUR BODY'S THIRST

Overview: You're Probably Not Drinking Enough

In 2013, 82 percent of Americans reported making a conscious effort to try to drink more water, rather than filling up on soft drinks and sweetened beverages. In fact, of all healthy habits people reported working on, drinking more water ranked #2 (with #1 being "eat more fruits and vegetables," which we'll cover in the next chapter).[9]

It's reassuring to hear that people are working on their health in such an important way, because our hydration levels have truly become an issue. Water alternatives line grocery store shelves everywhere, and we're drinking less and less water, on average. Studies show that 75 percent of Americans are chronically dehydrated.[10] 75 percent! The majority of Americans are so dehydrated, in fact, that they no longer feel the effects of dehydration. Our bodies eventually stop giving us signals of dehydration if we ignore the signals repeatedly. But I assure you that our overall health is still compromised if we are not adequately hydrated.

Quite often, when new clients share their health goals or discuss a problem they're experiencing, the first question that I'll ask is how much water they're currently drinking each day. Most people are quick to say they drink plenty of water, or that water can*NOT* be the issue. But once I remind them of the 75 percent statistic, it seems all the more plausible. Although increasing your water intake sounds like an overly simple concept to start out this book, I truly believe that almost everyone would be healthier if they drank more water.

The Health Benefits of Water

I could write an entire book about the many health benefits of water (and there are several already out there!) – its importance cannot be overemphasized. Maintaining adequate hydration levels is critical to dozens of functions in your body, including proper organ function, clear skin, optimal digestion, and healthy joints. Not drinking enough water can lead to "brain fog," migraines, skin breakouts, cravings, bad breath, and so much more.[11]

When I am dehydrated, I tend to get a throbbing headache at the nape of my neck and the front of my forehead, but symptoms vary dramatically by person. Maybe you feel the afternoon slump, can't shake cravings for sweets, wake up in the middle of the night with foot or leg cramps, or have problematic acne. These are just some of the immediate problems that could occur along with dehydration.

Common instantaneous signs of dehydration include fatigue, headache, cramping, bad mood, poor athletic performance, sugar cravings, unexplained hunger, and constipation. In the longer term, adequate hydration leads to such benefits as helping to lower cholesterol, lowering blood pressure, reducing the risk of digestive diseases, and facilitating weight loss or weight maintenance.

In the following sections, I'll highlight a few of these benefits and explain how healthy hydration levels can facilitate these positive changes. I'll discuss how hydration impacts cravings, fatigue, weight loss, and cholesterol levels. But if you're less concerned with how this actually works in the body, feel free to skip these four sections. We'll wrap the chapter up by discussing how to determine the right amount of water for your body, and how to reach your hydration goals once you set them.

Hydration and Cravings

So many of us experience cravings, and there are dozens of potential causes – from hormonal imbalances to nutrient deficiencies; from unsatisfying or unbalanced meals to a high-sugar diet. But, did you know that one often-overlooked potential cause of cravings is dehydration?

Thirst is so often confused with hunger. The signals our bodies send us are similar (including fatigue, stomach grumbling, and headaches), and most of us interpret those signals to mean we need food, rather than first trying water. However, if we eat when we're really thirsty, we may just be making the problem worse! Digestion is one of the many bodily functions that require water (to create digestive juices, and facilitate the movement of the food), so we wind up in a vicious cycle of needing more and more water, and making the problem even worse.

Hydration and Fatigue

Just as dehydration can cause hunger and cravings, it also can cause fatigue. Dr. Woodson Merrell of New York's Beth Israel Medical Center reported, "Half of the people who come to me complaining of fatigue are actually dehydrated."[12] The University of Rochester Medical Center reports that a loss of 1 percent of your body weight due to dehydration can cause decreased physical performance and feelings of fatigue, and a loss of just 2 percent to 4 percent can impact your mental functioning.[13]

The major reason we feel fatigued when we are dehydrated is that our bodies have to work overtime to conduct their standard functions and processes. When we are dehydrated, our blood volume is decreased (blood is over 80 percent water, and when the body overall does not have enough water, it pulls from the blood first). With lower blood volume, the body has to work harder to pump blood throughout the body. It is also more difficult to excrete toxins by urination, defecation, and perspiration. Even routine tasks like maintaining bodily temperature become harder. All of this extra effort may cause us to feel fatigued, even as we go about a routine day.

Dehydration also can slow down enzymes that help produce the body's energy. Our body's enzymes operate best in cells that are hydrated, but as we become dehydrated, some water is pulled from the cell to support the body's critical functions.[14] This causes us to feel fatigued, apathetic, and moody. However, there's good news! This can be very quickly reversed. Most people experience increased energy within a few hours of rehydrating with a lot of water. I have many clients who have noticed significant improvements in their day-to-day energy after they started drinking water consistently for just a few days.

Hydration and Weight Loss

We've discussed that dehydration leads to cravings, so eliminating those cravings by adequately hydrating is an obvious way to encourage weight loss with water. When we don't have false symptoms of hunger that are satisfied with unneeded food, we generally eat according to what our body really needs. And our bodies are remarkably good at maintaining optimal body weight – if only we can listen to the signals they give us.

You may have heard the suggestion to drink a large glass of water before eating a meal, and this stems from similar principles. Our stomachs can stretch, but they can only stretch so far. So if we drink water first, we already start the meal a bit "full" and can better gauge our body's signals of fullness and satiation. Some people report digestive difficulty when drinking large quantities of water before a meal, so I recommend experimenting with your own body before committing to this. If it helps you stop eating when you feel satisfied but not overly full, does not cause discomfort, and improves hydration, it is something I support.

In the section on "Hydration and Fatigue," we said being dehydrated slows down the activity of enzymes in our bodies. Enzymes also are used in metabolizing our food, and so our metabolism and fat burning can slow down if we lack sufficient hydration levels. The *Journal of Clinical Endocrinology & Metabolism* reported on a study that showed water drinking to increase the metabolic rate by almost 30 percent for a short time after drinking water.[15] Although the study was small, it showed that the potential added calorie expenditure from drinking more water may result in up to five pounds of weight loss per year.

Finally, water can increase weight loss by reducing symptoms of constipation. Water is absorbed through the walls of the colon before we excrete waste. In cases where we are dehydrated, too much water is pulled out of the colon (since the body needs it for other more important functions), and the stool becomes dry and difficult to eliminate. Not only does this sound unpleasant, it's also rough on your entire digestive system and could potentially cause you to retain excess weight.

Hydration and Cholesterol

With the proliferation of prescription medications that aim to lower cholesterol today, you may be surprised to learn that something as simple as drinking more water can help lower cholesterol. I have seen it time and time again in clients, many of whom promised me initially that their high cholesterol levels were "just genetic" or were impossible to lower without medication. At my urging, they begin hydrating consistently and improving their diets, and their cholesterol levels dropped to the acceptable ranges in just a few months.

The body is constantly prioritizing all bodily functions, and tries to conserve water for the most critical functions that keep us alive. One of the places that water is pulled from when the body senses dehydration is the intracellular fluid of the cells. When this happens, our bodies actually make more cholesterol to try to keep the water in the cells. This raises the cholesterol in the blood as well. Just by increasing our water intake, we can make a positive impact on our cholesterol levels, without actually changing what we are eating.

How Much Is Enough?

The most common advice says that we need 8 glasses of water (or 64 ounces) per day. Other recommendations suggest about 100 ounces for men and about 70 ounces for women. A third common suggestion is to take your body weight in pounds, divide by two, and drink that number of ounces of water (so, a 150-pound person would require 75 ounces of water). For a customized calculation using some of these methods, download The Lyons' Share's app, called *Drink More Water: 30-Day Challenge*, available in the iTunes store (just search for "The Lyons' Share water").

These calculation methods are all great starting places to give you an idea of how much water you need to consume. Still, the concept of bioindividuality applies to water just as it does to food, and we often need some experimentation to determine how much water our own bodies require. Thus, the "right" amount of water varies dramatically by person, and even by day ... the right amount for you depends on your level of exercise, the temperature and altitude, your unique body composition, what you're eating (processed and salty foods require more water to digest) and your hydrating food intake (fruits, vegetables, and soups all contain water, which can add up and lessen the amount of pure water you need to drink).

If you truly want to gauge your hydration levels, the color of your urine is the best way to do so. There are several color charts available online, including one on The Lyons' Share website.[16] Don't worry – I'm not suggesting that you carry around a chart everywhere you go, but it's helpful to take a quick glance to know if you need to boost your water intake. You should aim for a pale yellow color, like light lemonade. Dark yellow or brownish-tinted urine is an immediate indicator of dehydration, so be sure to hydrate adequately if you see that. Some vitamins and supplements can change the color of your urine, so if you're taking supplements, pay attention to any *change* in color, which may indicate dehydration.

Many of my clients wonder if they're at risk of drinking too much water. Yes, this is possible – in fact, overhydration can cause a dangerous condition called hyponatremia. However, this is rare for otherwise healthy individuals, and you'd have to be drinking a *ton* of water to bring about this problem. I frequently drink more than 120 ounces a day, and I am not worried about this issue. If you are concerned that you are drinking too much water, I recommend seeing a doctor to get your electrolyte levels checked.

What "Counts" as Water?

Although we often hear that we need to drink "fluids," this does not mean anything in liquid form. You've probably guessed that soda does not "count" as water when you're working on your hydration levels.

Here's an interesting (and depressing) statistic: in 1998, Americans averaged 54 gallons of soda per person, and only 42 gallons of water![17] (Today, we've improved to 44 gallons of soda and 58 gallons of water, which still leaves significant room for improvement!). If you can't get by without your soda, I'd recommend alternating one glass of soda with one glass of water, or making sure you consume the two side-by-side. Or, try club soda or naturally flavored sparkling water (I like the brand called La Croix), both calorie-free and tasty ways to get your fix of fizz.

Fruits, vegetables, and broth-based soups also contain water, and contribute to your hydration levels. Although it's nearly impossible to add up the ounces of pure water you're getting from every piece of produce you eat, keep in mind that your needs for pure drinking water may be slightly decreased if you eat large amounts of fruits, vegetables, or soups.

Juice, milk, and coconut water also contribute to your overall hydration, although I don't recommend using these as a substitute for all of your plain drinking water. The calories and sugar content can add up quickly, so while they may be complements to your water intake, they should not replace it.

Sports drinks can also be used to quench thirst and contribute to hydration. However, I believe sports drinks (like Gatorade and Powerade) are heavily overused by the casual exerciser. If you're going out for a 20-minute walk in cool temperatures, first, congratulations!, but second, you do NOT need to down a monster-sized Gatorade. Your body is capable of restoring your electrolyte balance by itself, as long as you're drinking regular water and eating a balanced diet. In general, I think sports drinks should be limited to exercise longer than an hour, at a medium- to high-intensity, and/or in hot conditions. For most other exercise, water should suffice!

If so many other beverages "count" toward your hydration, do coffee and wine "count" as well? Not so fast. Recent research suggests that coffee is not actually as dehydrating as we once thought (aside from a very mild diuretic effect), so there's no reason to avoid it altogether if you're concerned about staying hydrated. Still, it doesn't hydrate us like plain and simple water, so it doesn't "count" for these purposes. I like to consider coffee and caffeinated tea as neutral when I'm calculating my own water intake, and I consider alcoholic beverages and soda as negative (meaning I need to drink more water to make up for any alcohol or soda I consume). Herbal tea is hydrating, so go ahead and count it towards your hydration goals!

How to Increase your Water Intake

If you're not drinking much water right now, the prospect of drinking 64 ounces or more per day may seem daunting. You may not like the taste of water, may not feel thirsty, or may just simply forget to drink because you're not in the habit.

If any of these describe you, I advise you to start slowly. Try to gauge how much water you're currently drinking per day. For the next week, increase that by 8 ounces. Continue increasing by 8 ounces each week until you reach a level that seems appropriate for your body (refer to the previous section called "How Much is Enough?" for guidance). Making small, incremental changes makes large dietary shifts seem more realistic than intimidating.

Here are a few additional ways to increase your water intake, and get into the habit of hydrating regularly:

- **ALWAYS CARRY A WATER BOTTLE WITH YOU.** Get a reusable bottle that you like, and keep it where you keep your wallet, keys, or other object that you don't usually leave home without. Keep another reusable bottle on your desk at work, and set a glass in an area of the house where you tend to relax. Simply having the water bottle with you at all times will increase your consumption naturally, since you don't have to go out of your way to remind yourself to drink.

- **INFUSE YOUR WATER WITH FLAVOR.** If you're a person who finds drinking plain water boring or tasteless, adding fruits, herbs, or vegetables to your water may help. Simply take a large pitcher, fill it with water and ice, and add a bit of flavor. I like adding several sliced cucumber and strawberries (as featured in this chapter's recipe). Experiment with other flavors as well: mint, ginger, lemon, orange, grapefruit, sliced grapes, pomegranate seeds, and peaches are other great options!

- **TRACK YOUR WATER INTAKE IN A WAY THAT WORKS FOR YOU.** When you're just starting out on your hydration journey, it's often helpful to track your intake for a few days, weeks, or even months. I help my clients determine a tracking method that doesn't seem burdensome and won't be forgotten. Some like to set out enough bottles to reach their water intake goal at the beginning of the day. If there are 5 bottles on your kitchen counter, and you know you must finish them before the day is over, you're more likely to start drinking early. Some like to use my "rubber band method" – put an appropriate number of rubber bands on your wrist each morning (depending on the size of your bottle and your hydration needs). Switch one from your wrist to your bottle each time you refill it. You must switch all the rubber bands by the end of the day! There are also some bottles with built-in tracking mechanisms: I like the reusable cup with a straw from AquaTally, which includes a rotating dial to track the number of daily refills.

- **KEEP A BOTTLE (OR BOTTLES) IN YOUR CAR.** Many of my clients spend a significant amount of time in the car (commuting, shuttling kids to activities, etc.), but don't always have water available to drink. By simply keeping an empty bottle in their car, they find themselves more likely to stop and fill it up, and are often surprised to report that they ended up drinking it during the car trip! I also recommend stashing a case of disposable water bottles in the trunk (unless you live in very hot temperatures) to have a constant supply for yourself and others!

- **DOWNLOAD AN APP.** I have created a Lyons' Share app called *Drink More Water*, which is a 30-day challenge that calculates a hydration target for your personal circumstances, sends three reminders a day to ensure that you're keeping up with your goal, and sends you daily health tips. You can find the app by searching for "The Lyons' Share water" in the iTunes store or visiting: https://itunes.apple.com/us/app/drink-more-water-30-day-challenge/id947445467

- **KEEP A GLASS OF WATER BY YOUR BED.** Drink it as soon as you wake up – we are most dehydrated in the morning, and our bodies crave water. Drinking a glass of pure water before you head straight to the coffee machine will work wonders on your energy levels and may reduce headaches, if you suffer regularly. Drinking water in the morning also flushes out toxins from the previous day.

- **TRY A CLEANSING WATER BEVERAGE IN THE MORNING.** To take your morning glass of water to the next level, try one of these two detoxifying combinations before you eat or drink anything else in the morning. For a soothing, relaxing start to the morning, drink a mug of warm or hot water with lemon slices. Or, for detoxification and digestive health, drink a glass of cold water with a few teaspoons of raw apple cider vinegar (I like the kind made by Bragg's, which is available in most grocery stores). Both of these may reduce cravings throughout the day, aid in detoxification, improve digestion, and otherwise contribute to hydration and health.

- **TRY DRINKING A GLASS OF WATER BEFORE EACH MEAL.** Some studies show that drinking a glass of water before each meal contributes to weight loss. In fact, one random-ized controlled trial showed a 44 percent greater decline in weight over a 12-week period for those who drank about 16 ounces of water versus those who did not drink water before their meal.[18] If you're trying to lose weight, drinking a glass before each meal may be a helpful reminder *and* may speed up your weight loss. As mentioned previously, if this causes you digestive distress, avoid it.

There's an added bonus to all this water: almost all of my soda-drinking clients who begin drinking more water have significantly reduced or eliminated their soda intake naturally! I rarely tell my clients to stop drinking soda, but rather tell them to start drinking water. Between feeling more energized, having fewer cravings, and feeling more full throughout the day, the desire for soda naturally drifts away!

~ Recipe: Strawberry-Cucumber Water ~

INGREDIENTS

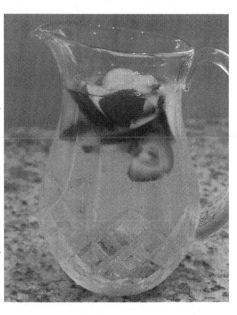

1 large pitcher of water

About ½ cup of fruit or vegetable slices of your choice

(optional): small pinch of salt

INSTRUCTIONS

Add four thinly-sliced strawberries and ½ cup of thinly
sliced cucumber to a large
pitcher. Although it sounds
strange, adding a small pinch of salt will often help the flavors
of the fruit stand out. Fill with water and ice. If you drink all the
water, feel free to continue refilling the pitcher (with strawberries and cucumber). The slices will last 1-2 days, as long as the
pitcher is refrigerated.

Don't forget!

To get the exclusive *Lyons' Share Healthy Pantry Guide,* download
the free bonuses to this book at www.StartHereBonus.com.

CHAPTER THREE

YOUR PARENTS WERE RIGHT!

"Eat your vegetables!"
"No dessert until you finish your broccoli!"
"Eating spinach will make you strong!"
"If you eat your carrots, you'll be able to see in the dark!"

If you've never heard any of these, you're either a rare child who devoured your vegetables unasked (your lucky parents!), or your parents gave up and stopped begging somewhere along the way. For centuries, we've been told that vegetables are healthy, are critical for kids (whether they like them or not), and should make up a portion of every meal. But have you ever stopped to wonder why vegetables are so good for you?

Overview: The Health Benefits of Vegetables

Think about any popular diet that has worked for you or someone you know. Low-fat, Weight Watchers, South Beach Diet, Paleo, the list goes on. As different as they may all be, they share one commonality. Almost every single diet that has actually produced weight loss or health results has included and emphasized vegetables. There aren't many nutrition practices that have withstood the test of time (we hear that egg yolks will kill you one day and save you the next), but vegetables have very rarely been blasphemed the way other food groups have been. And there are good reasons for this!

The fiber, antioxidants, and phytonutrients in vegetables exist in such an ideal ratio that there is no other food group as rich in naturally occurring nutrients with so few calories. Eating a variety of fruits and vegetables is a more effective way to ensure your nutrient requirements are met than any multivitamin or other treatment on the market. They fill you up, help your digestion, give you energy, and promote long-term health.

The USDA reports that consuming an overall healthy diet that is rich in fruits and vegetables may reduce risk for heart disease, including heart attack and stroke, as well as many types of cancers.[19] Other studies have shown a clear correlation between incidence of cancer in those who eat diets higher in processed foods, refined grains, and meat, and lower in fruits and vegetables. In fact, a 2012 Anticancer Research report claimed that over 30 percent of adult cancers can be delayed or prevented with proper nutrition, exercise, and body weight, and that vegetables are a major component of this prevention.[20] Fiber has been linked to lower LDL ("bad") cholesterol, more stable blood sugar levels, and lower rates of metabolic syndrome, obesity, and diabetes.

There are many reasons to eat your vegetables, but I'll highlight just a few (fiber, antioxidants, and phytonutrients) in the next few sections, then share my "VEGGIES" strategies to increase the quantity and quality of vegetables in your diet.

Fiber

One major reason vegetables are so healthy is that they are rich in fiber. Of the recommended 25 grams (g) a day for women and 38 grams a day for men (and I often recommend even more, depending on the person!), the average American eats only 15 grams of fiber a day[21]. This is probably because the standard American diet is so low in vegetables, which are one of the best sources of fiber available.

So, why does it matter that we're lacking in this regard? First, fibrous food is more filling, which may prevent you from overeating later in the day and help you feel satisfied on fewer calories. When fiber sits in your digestive system, it absorbs water and can even expand, helping to "clear out" your digestive system more quickly. Basically, fiber can help keep you regular and can prevent you from becoming constipated. I think we can all agree that is a good thing!

Getting your recommended dosage of fiber won't happen from just adding a leaf of lettuce to your cheeseburger. A half-cup serving of green peas, sweet potato, or Brussels sprouts will each contain 4g (with relatively few calories and loads of nutrients). Beans can also help, with around 6g per half-cup, and whole grain-based cereals generally have about 2-3g per serving. Most fruits also have about 2g per serving. Remember what I discussed in the introduction to this book: When you're eating healthy, nutrient-dense food, you can consume a lot of it!

Antioxidants and Phytonutrients

Vegetables (and fruits) are also packed with antioxidants, making them powerhouses for fighting disease and inflammation. Antioxidants counteract a process called oxidation in your body's cells, which occurs naturally from aging, exercising, breathing in, or consuming toxins ... basically, just living our daily lives.

All of these activities produce "free radicals," which are harmful to our bodies, and antioxidants get rid of free radicals. If all of that sounded confusing to you, suffice it to say that antioxidants prevent damage to your cells, and may help prevent chronic diseases such as cancer, heart disease, and stroke. Antioxidants common in the foods we eat include vitamin C, vitamin E, and beta-carotene.

The wonderful thing about fruits and vegetables is that antioxidants are present in perfect combinations to combat disease. For example, spinach and other leafy greens contain high quantities of vitamins A, C, K, lutein, manganese, as well as fiber, iron, and folate. Diets high in spinach have been shown to protect against stroke, coronary heart disease, age-related macular degeneration, and cataracts, and to support immune function.

Vegetables and fruits (as well as whole grains, nuts, beans, and tea) also contain a huge variety of phytonutrients, which also help prevent disease and keep your body working properly. Phytonutrients are a broader category than antioxidants, and some phytonutrients are also antioxidants. In fact, there are more than 2,000 phytonutrients present in plant foods!

Just like antioxidants, the phytonutrients in plant foods are available in combinations that are efficiently used by our bodies. This means that taking phytonutrient supplements often does not show the same disease-fighting benefits that consuming actual fruits and vegetables does. You may know that oranges are rich in vitamin C, for example, and you may have heard that vitamin C is good for your immune system. So, you take a vitamin C supplement, which claims to have 1,000 percent or more of your recommended daily allowance for vitamin C. This sounds more powerful than eating an orange, which has about 100 percent of your RDA for vitamin C.

What you're missing, though, is the thousands of other antioxidants, phytonutrients, and healthful components that the orange contains, but that the supplement lacks. Your body simply doesn't absorb an artificial source of vitamin C as well as it absorbs the real deal!

In general, consuming a wide range of foods like berries, cherries, leafy greens, tomatoes, broccoli, and other fruits and vegetables is the best way to ensure you take in the antioxidants and phytonutrients your body needs to prevent disease.

Overview: VEGGIES

I created the acronym "VEGGIES" to help my health coaching clients increase the quantity and quality of vegetables in their diets. It's a handy little reminder, and great to print out and stick to your refrigerator, put in your wallet, or post in another place where you'll frequently see it.

V: *Variety is key ... eat the rainbow!*

We often identify the different phytonutrients in foods by the color of those foods. For example, carotenoids and lycopene are present in red and orange foods, like carrots, cantaloupe, oranges, pumpkin, sweet potatoes, tomatoes, and watermelon. These phytonutrients help prevent cancer and improve immunity. Flavenoids and phenols are present in deep red and purple foods, like berries, red grapes, red wine, dark chocolate, and citrus. These phytonutrients help lower cholesterol and prevent heart disease. Cruciferous vegetables like broccoli, cauliflower, and Brussels sprouts are rich in polyphenols that support cardiovascular health, immune function, and cancer risk reduction.

Because each color of vegetables and fruits has different benefits, it's important to try to include many different colors every day, or at least throughout the week. Can you challenge yourself to get at least one item from each color this week? Make it a game with your kids, and have them keep track of each color they eat.

Here are a few ideas for each color:

RED: apples, cherries, strawberries, cranberries, grapefruit, pomegranates, raspberries, watermelon, beets, red peppers, radishes, red cabbage, red onions, red potatoes, tomatoes.

ORANGE: apricots, cantaloupe, mango, nectarines, oranges, papaya, peaches, tangerines, butternut squash, carrots, pumpkin.

YELLOW: lemons, yellow pears, pineapple, yellow peppers, summer squash, corn.

GREEN: avocado, green apples, green grapes, honeydew, kiwi, limes, green peas, artichokes, arugula, asparagus, broccoli, Brussels sprouts, green beans, cabbage, celery, cucumbers, kale, leafy greens, lettuce, green onions, okra, green peppers, snow peas, spinach, snap peas, watercress, zucchini.

BLUE: blueberries, blue potatoes.

PURPLE: blackberries, purple grapes, plums, figs, eggplant, purple cauliflower, purple asparagus, purple carrots.

WHITE: bananas, white peaches, white nectarines, cauliflower, garlic, onions, jicama, kohlrabi, parsnips, turnips.

I am thrilled when clients increase their intake of *any* vegetables, but still try to guide them toward the healthiest versions. I recommend consuming unlimited amounts of leafy greens and brightly-colored non-starchy vegetables (like peppers, broccoli, green beans, and asparagus), and limiting starchy vegetables (like potatoes, corn, peas, and starchy squashes) to a serving or two per day.

E: Experiment with different cooking methods

If I had a glass of water for every time I've heard someone tell me that they hate Brussels sprouts, I certainly wouldn't need to worry about my hydration levels! Whenever anyone says that to me, though, I always ask how the Brussels sprouts they've eaten have been prepared, and almost inevitably, they recollect the boiled Brussels sprouts their mothers forced them to eat at the childhood dinner table. I am hard-pressed to think of *any* vegetable that is more delicious when boiled, so I don't blame the person for not liking their boiled sprouts. Incidentally, boiling is not usually the healthiest option either, as many of the nutrients are leached from the vegetables and lost in the boiling water.

I encourage you to experiment with different cooking methods to find the ones that you enjoy with each vegetable. I find that I love most vegetables roasted in the oven – I simply pre-heat it to 400 degrees, spread the chopped vegetables on a foil-lined baking sheet sprayed with olive oil or cooking spray, cover them with one more spray of olive oil or cooking spray and a bit of seasoning (simple salt and pepper always works, or I experiment with cayenne, basil, oregano, paprika, Italian seasoning, or any variety of other spice or herb!), and bake for 17-22 minutes, depending on the vegetable. This method is fast and easy, and also caramelizes the vegetables to bring out the delicious flavors!

If you don't want to roast your vegetables, or if you're dining in a restaurant, I encourage you to go for boiled, broiled, grilled, roasted, baked, lightly sautéed, steamed, or raw. These methods are almost always healthier than others (indicated by words like "fried," "crispy," "crunchy," or "creamy"). Experiment to find what you prefer – I love grilled asparagus and peppers, quick-boiled green beans, roasted broccoli and Brussels sprouts, sautéed spinach and chard, raw snap peas, and steamed zucchini.

G: Go to the Farmer's Market

I love supporting my Farmer's Market, and do so at every opportunity I get. Here are my top 7 reasons to go to your Farmer's Market:

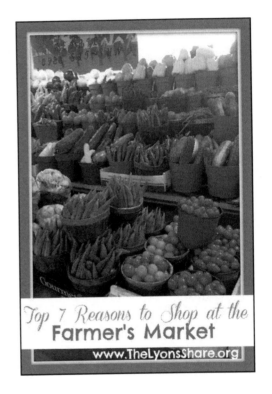

YOU WILL SUPPORT LOCAL FARMERS AND BUSINESSES: This is the most common reason for shopping at the Farmer's Markets. When you see the farmers in person and have a conversation with them, it's hard not to want to support their hard work. Small farms require a ton of manual labor, are often unsubsidized, and are subject to a lot of volatility (weather, pests, demand, competition, etc.). Every little bit of support we can give back to the small, local farmers helps!

YOU'RE MORE LIKELY TO BE EXCITED ABOUT EATING FRUITS AND VEGETABLES: By nature, we are more likely to eat what is in plain sight in our kitchens, and I encourage you to keep a variety of fruits and vegetables on your kitchen counters and in visible places in your refrigerator. What better way to feel excited about the fruits and vegetables that are available to you than to shop for them yourself at the Farmer's Market? Just by going to the effort of getting there, walking through the stalls, and picking out your produce, I can almost guarantee that you'll feel more motivated to eat it! This tip works for your kids, too.

IT'S OFTEN CHEAPER TO BUY ORGANIC PRODUCE AT THE FARMER'S MARKET: You may think that organic produce is more expensive than conventional, but at the Farmer's Market, I often find it sold for less than what I'd have to pay at my local grocery store (especially if I am buying local and seasonal items). It also helps to talk to the farmers or sellers – many farms grow their food "organically" (without chemicals or artificial fertilizers/pesticides), but cannot afford to be USDA certified and receive the official organic label. Use your judgment here, but I still feel great about buying this produce.

IT'S MORE ENVIRONMENTALLY SUSTAINABLE: True – some stands at the Farmer's Market actually buy imported produce from wholesalers, but in general, a lot of the produce at the Farmer's Market has traveled less distance than the produce found in grocery stores, making it friendlier to the environment. Did you know that the average American meal travels 1,500+ miles to arrive on your plate? Shopping at Farmer's Markets reduces that distance by a significant amount.[22]

IT'S A FUN WAY TO TEACH YOUR KIDS (OR LEARN YOURSELF!) ABOUT THE GROWING PROCESS: Most of the farmers I talk to are very open to explaining the growing process, or teaching me more about the produce. What a fun way to educate your kids during the summer and get them excited about healthy foods!

YOU GET A FREE SNACK: I know this one sounds a little trite, but I honestly look forward to the samples at the Farmer's Market every single time! The sellers will put out samples of their best-tasting produce, so the bites you get are absolutely delicious. Cucumber slices, tomatoes sprinkled with sea salt, jicama with cayenne, freshly sliced pineapple, oranges, berries, you name it – I love all the samples!

YOU'RE MORE LIKELY TO BUY SEASONAL PRODUCE, AND A WIDER VARIETY OF PRODUCE: Even if seasonal produce is available, we tend to get into a routine in the grocery store - buying the same produce items week after week. When we see the bright colors, beautiful displays, and interesting layouts at the Farmer's Market, though, we are more likely to be attracted to the seasonal (nutrient-rich!) produce, as well as to step out of our comfort zones and try new varieties of produce.

G: Go Organic (at least for the Dirty Dozen)

Agricultural technology has produced countless advances that make it possible to feed a growing world population with fewer farmers. Sounds great, right? It is a wonderful thing ... at least on the surface. The problem is that many of these technological advances are injecting so many chemicals, fertilizers, and preservatives into our food supply. The advances are occurring so quickly that research cannot keep up to determine whether our health is at risk.

You've probably seen labels in your local grocery store that differentiate "organic" and "conventional" fruits and vegetables. You may even have thought they must have done something special to the "organic" produce to make it better for you (and more expensive!). But think about the food that your grandmother ate growing up. Do you think she had an "organic" or a "conventional" label on her carrots? No! They were just carrots! They were grown without the plethora of chemicals used today, and our bodies recognized them as food, not foreign substances.

"Organic" refers to how produce is grown, and the FDA regulates usage of the label. Produce labeled "organic" is produced, grown, and harvested without most conventional pesticides, fertilizers made with synthetic ingredients, bioengineering, or ionizing radiation. Natural fertilizers like manure and compost may still be used, and pests and weeds must be managed without synthetic herbicides and insecticides.

Similarly, an "organic" label on meat means the animal was raised without growth-promoting hormones or antibiotics. Food products labeled "100 percent organic" must be made with ingredients that are at least 95 percent organic, and food products labeled "organic" must be made with ingredients that are at least 70 percent organic (and if that seems a bit misleading, I agree with you. But that's a topic for another entire book!).

So now that you understand what the label means, should you care about this label? I would argue that yes, you should, at least in a handful of cases. Not only does organic farming reduce pollution and environmental damage, but the impact on our health seems highly favorable.

It's worth noting that the actual nutrition content may not be significantly different in organic or conventional produce. Some studies report that organically-grown produce contains more nutrients,[23] and others show no difference,[24] so I won't jump to any conclusions here. But it's not the nutrient content I'm worried about in this debate – it's all the extra stuff I'm getting from conventional produce that I'd rather avoid.

Two-thirds of produce samples in government tests showed pesticide residues.[25] There are numerous laboratory studies showing that pesticides can be linked to health problems such as birth defects, nerve damage, cancer, and many more chronic diseases.[26] At the same time, though, the federal government currently allows pesticides to be used, and has tests that show small doses of the chemicals are not harmful to human health. They say they are managing the amount of pesticides used so there is "reasonable certainty they will pose no harm."[27]

But do you know what? Less than 7 percent of the chemicals used in high volume in our food supply have been heavily tested, and we don't have tests showing the impact of repeated exposure to so many chemicals in combination. We can be pretty sure that we are exposed to **a lot** of chemicals – in fact, there are over 75,000 synthetic chemicals in circulation, and they're constantly entering our bodies through our skin, eyes, mouth, nose, and – of course – the food we eat.

And remember their purpose – many of them are designed to kill pests, so they're very toxic! At least 76 million birds are killed annually by pesticides, and even though my body is bigger and stronger than a bird's body, it's a statistic staggering enough to convince me that I don't want high doses of those chemicals in my body if I can avoid them.

So, scare tactics aside, what do we do about it?

I recommend starting with the "Dirty Dozen" and commit to buying organic versions of the vegetables and fruits on the list. The Dirty Dozen is published yearly by the Environmental Working Group, listing the 12 vegetables and fruits that are most likely to be contaminated by pesticides. For 2015, the list included:[28]

For these items, I would highly recommend shifting to organic. Yes, I understand that organic produce is more expensive, and I also understand that these may be some of your favorite items! Could you choose one or two items every month, and commit to switching to organic for those items only? The impact on your budget will be only a few dollars a month, and I assure you your health is worth it.

If the switch to organic is just not realistic, try to switch your consumption to other items. If you are used to packing an apple with lunch every day, how about an orange? If you regularly buy potatoes, how about sweet potatoes instead? If you're a sucker for berries as I am, the organic versions are far cheaper when bought frozen, and often can be found on sale.

By the way, if you're reading closely, you'll notice that there are 14 items, not 12 ... the EWG expanded its list, but wanted to keep the catchy "Dirty Dozen" title.

Here's some good news: the EWG also publishes the "Clean Fifteen," which are the fifteen *least* contaminated vegetables and fruits. For these items, you can save your money! Their thick skin, method of growth, or genetic makeup makes them resistant to pesticides, so the conventional items won't do you harm.

For 2015, this list included:

- *Asparagus*
- *Avocados*
- *Cabbage*
- *Canteloupe*
- *Cauliflower*
- *Eggplant*
- *Grapefruit*
- *Kiwi*
- *Mangoes*
- *Onions*
- *Papayas*
- *Pineapples*
- *Sweet peas (frozen)*
- *Sweet potatoes*

In the end, I certainly would rather you eat conventional vegetables and fruits than no vegetables and fruits at all. Our bodies are remarkably good at fighting off foreign invaders like pesticides, and the benefits of all that extra nutrition will almost always outweigh the risks of pesticides. But, if you can make it work, why not give yourself a fighting chance at your very best health by choosing organic for the 14 items listed in the Dirty Dozen?

I: Instead of an appetizer, choose a salad

Eating at restaurants can be convenient, quick, and fun, but can also quickly derail our health goals. Did you know the average restaurant meal contains 2-3 times the estimated calorie needs of an adult at a single meal?[29] Some restaurant meals even top 3,000 calories, which is far more than most adults need in a day!

One of the main reasons that eating at restaurants is less healthy is that we tend to eat larger quantities of food. Think about this: At home, you probably wouldn't prepare yourself an appetizer, a bread basket, an entrée, and a dessert, right? I discuss more strategies to manage restaurants healthily in Chapter Six, but one simple way to cut back on the additional calories at restaurants is to choose a salad to start your meal instead of a heavy appetizer.

Starting with a simple salad (preferably with a light dressing or a drizzle of balsamic and olive oil) is a great way to fit in extra vegetables, and fill your stomach a bit so you won't overeat.

E: Expand your horizons ... try new varieties!

Another common reason my clients tell me they don't eat vegetables is because they are bored with the two or three varieties they know how to prepare, or they've only ever eaten canned green beans and mushy steamed broccoli. I can't blame them for disliking those boring varieties!

I always recommend that people who are new to their health journeys experiment by trying one new vegetable each week. There are thousands of types of vegetables in the world, and just because you don't enjoy one variety does not mean you don't enjoy vegetables overall ... you need to keep trying!

If you've never had roasted okra, shaved kohlrabi on a salad, fresh jicama sticks as a snack, dehydrated kale chips, sweet potato fries, or zucchini noodles, you still have some experimenting to do! Make it fun – allow your children to pick out a new variety they see at the Farmer's Market, or try to choose a new color of vegetable that they want to enjoy each week. Don't get discouraged if there is one variety or method of preparation that isn't your favorite ... I firmly believe that *everyone* can find some kind of vegetable they enjoy!

S: Sneak them in (to smoothies, soups, and more)

Many of my clients tell me they just don't like vegetables, or their kids are turned off by seeing vegetables on their plates. Of course, in a perfect scenario, we all would enjoy eating vegetables in their natural forms, but I understand this isn't a reality for many people.

In these situations, I encourage sneaking in vegetables wherever possible, at least at the beginning. Many people are opposed to the idea of "fooling" their children into eating vegetables, or don't favor the concept of covering up the flavor, but I think it's a great place to start. I have heard numerous stories of children who begin eating some form of vegetables (or begin taking antioxidant-rich supplements made from fruits and vegetables) who end up craving more healthy foods, and opening their palates to a variety of fruits and vegetables they wouldn't have touched before. For this reason, along with the fact that our bodies truly need the nutrients from fruits and vegetables, I'm not opposed to sneaking in vegetables, and often encourage my clients to do so.

A few of my favorite ways to sneak in vegetables include smoothies, soups and stews, pasta substitutes, mashed potato substitutes, egg scrambles and egg muffins, and even baked goods.

SMOOTHIES: I very rarely make a smoothie without adding in a hefty dose of greens. Some of my favorites include spinach, kale, cucumber, celery, and even zucchini or broccoli! I am so used to seeing green-tinted smoothies that I don't bat an eye upon seeing them. But for those who are more skeptical, I recommend flavoring the smoothie with mint. Mint chocolate chip ice cream is often green, so a green-tinted mint smoothie doesn't seem so off-putting to many. My recipe for "Summer RefreshMINT Smoothie," a great way to sneak in some leafy greens in a delicious and healthy smoothie, is included at the end of this chapter.

SOUPS AND STEWS: I also recommend making veggie-filled soups or stews for two reasons. One, people tend to be more open to consuming vegetables when they're chopped into fine pieces and masked within a soup or stew. Two, they're a fantastic way to be prepared for busy situations. If you make a large pot of soup at the beginning of the week, you can refrigerate individual portions and have healthy, hearty meals ready to go when you walk into your home. They're also great to freeze (again, in individual portions) so that you have something to defrost when you arrive back in town or come home late. We've all had those moments of staring into the refrigerator and aimlessly thinking about what we could eat; having frozen portions of healthy soup can put an end to this aimless staring. My recipe for Healthy 10-Minute Tortilla Soup is included at the end of this chapter.

PASTA SUBSTITUTES: Did you know that vegetables make great pasta substitutes? A tool called a "spiralizer" can easily shred vegetables like zucchini, squash, or sweet potatoes into pasta-like strands, which you can boil for a few minutes and serve as you would pasta. Spaghetti squash also is a great substitute for pasta, and allows those watching their waistlines to eat a large quantity of "comfort food" without packing on the extra calories in a bowl of pasta. Even shredded broccoli slaw or cabbage (sold as cole slaw without the dressing) can be a great addition to soups and stews, and somewhat resembles small noodles when cooked. My recipe for "Sizzlin' Southwestern Spaghetti Squash" is included at the end of this chapter.

MASHED POTATO SUBSTITUTES: I knew that mashed potatoes were a great way to hide vegetables when I tried my mashed cauliflower recipe on my dad, who isn't the biggest fan of vegetables in their purest form. Vegetables like cauliflower, parsnips, and rutabaga can be pureed and masked as potatoes without anyone batting an eye, and are great "hidden veggies" for those who generally don't like vegetables. My recipe for "Just Like Mom's Chunky Mashed Cauliflower" is included at the end of this chapter.

EGG SCRAMBLES AND EGG MUFFINS: As a runner, I'm always conscious of refueling my body with a balanced meal after I exert myself with exercise. One of my go-to favorite meals is a large egg scramble, topped with salsa and avocado or a sprinkle of parmesan cheese. Not only are egg scrambles simple to prepare, they are a great way to use up any extra vegetables you have on hand. Simply sauté 1-2 cups of chopped vegetables in a large skillet, and add in your choice of eggs. I generally use one to two whole eggs and two egg whites. Feel free to experiment with your own choice of vegetables – broccoli, cauliflower, zucchini, squash, parsnips, sweet potatoes, broccoli slaw, spinach, kale, and mushrooms are some of my favorites.

Another way I frequently enjoy eggs is in "egg muffins." I often make these at the beginning of a busy week, and store them in the refrigerator for quick, nutritious, grab-and-go breakfast options. You can even freeze the muffins to ensure that you have healthy choices on hand on the busiest of days. A recipe for Grab-and-Go Egg Muffins is included at the end of this chapter.

BAKED GOODS: If you want to get adventurous, you can even sneak vegetables into baked goods. Zucchini, carrots, pumpkin, and sweet potatoes are probably the easiest to start with, as their flavors are easily masked by other ingredients in the dish, and their textures are easy to work with. You can try substituting these ingredients in any of your favorite recipes. Here are a few healthy baking substitutions that I use regularly:

- Substitute ¼-cup of canned pumpkin puree (not pumpkin pie filling, which has lots of extra sugar) for each egg called for in a recipe.

- Substitute an equal amount of pumpkin puree for the oil called for in a recipe.

- Substitute an equal amount of unsweetened applesauce for the oil or butter called for in a recipe.

- Substitute an equal amount of mashed banana for the oil or butter called for in a recipe.

- Substitute Greek yogurt for sour cream or mayonnaise, or add a bit of Greek yogurt to keep your healthier baked goods moist.

- Substitute one can of black beans, rinsed, drained, and mashed, for 1 cup of flour.

- Choose whole grain or nut-based flours. I like quinoa flour, almond meal, oat flour, and standard 100 percent whole wheat flour. My recipe for "Zucchini Apple Breakfast Muffins" is included at the end of Chapter Four.

SUPPLEMENTS: As mentioned, I have seen many examples of picky kids who previously did not eat any vegetables at all turning to a high-quality supplement, and seeing dramatic improvements. For this reason, I recommend greens supplements to several of my clients, both adults and children, as a way to "bridge the gap" between what they need and what they ingest. Two products I like are Amazing Grass (available from Amazon or other retailers, at most health food stores) and Juice Plus+. Despite eating about 12 servings of vegetables a day consistently, I take a small dose of Juice Plus+ each day, and carry Amazing Grass when traveling, because I'm convinced that the very best way to prevent long-term chronic disease is to have as high an influx of antioxidants as possible.

Let's be clear, I will always think the best way to get our nutrients is directly from fruits and vegetables. But ... kids need at least five fist-sized servings of vegetables and fruits a day, and adults need 8-13. In the crazy busy world we live in today, so many people just don't get that.

After taking Juice Plus+, more than 70 percent of kids miss fewer days of school, 70 percent take fewer prescription medicines, 76 percent end up eating MORE fruits and vegetables (because their body starts "craving" the nutrients once they are introduced). Of course, the nutrients are also critical for long-term health, so the Juice Plus+ supplements are a good way to make sure the kids are getting those nutrients even on days they're not eating all the vegetables they should.

Should you be interested in trying Juice Plus+ for yourself or your family, you can order directly from my website, www.meganlyons. juiceplus.com, or email me directly at megan@thelyonsshare.org.

~ Recipe: An Ugly Secret ~

This is my absolute favorite last-minute "I-have-no-energy-to-think-about-making-a-real-recipe-but-I-still-want-something-healthy-and-quick meal." And the good news is that you can customize it to fit your nutritional needs, taste preferences, and what you have in your fridge/freezer. It's very healthy, and very filling ... and a great way to get in a few servings of vegetables!

Makes 1 serving. Nutrition information will depend on vegetables and protein source used.

INSTRUCTIONS

Preheat oven to 400 degrees.

While oven is heating, chop your choice of vegetables into bite-sized pieces. I love using broccoli slaw in this dish, as well as broccoli, cauliflower, eggplant, Brussels sprouts, mushrooms, zucchini, squash, green beans, asparagus, okra, onions, or any other vegetables I have on hand! You want about 2 cups of chopped vegetables per serving.

Spray a foil-lined baking pan with cooking spray or olive oil. Spread on your chopped vegetables, and roast for 15-20 minutes (depending on the strength of your oven), or until just beginning to brown.

Cook a source of lean protein (options may include a vegetable burger, chicken breast, canned tuna or salmon, tofu, beans, lean steak).

Put everything in a large bowl, add some tomato sauce (choose the kind with no added sugar, and opt for low-sodium and organic if available), and stir.

Top with Parmesan cheese or nutritional yeast and enjoy!

~ Recipe: Healthy 10-Minute Tortilla Soup ~

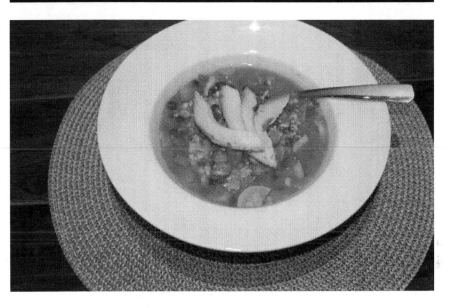

I don't think I've ever met someone who doesn't love the comforting flavor of tortilla soup, and you don't have to sacrifice the taste if you don't want the calorie-laden restaurant versions. Enjoy this veggie- and protein-packed version straight from the comfort of your own home!

Makes 6 servings (and tastes great after being frozen! Just portion into individual containers, freeze, and defrost when you need a quick and convenient meal). Each serving contains 240 calories, 6g fat, 24g carbs, and 23g protein.

INGREDIENTS

20 ounces 99 percent lean ground turkey

1 can diced tomatoes

1 can black beans, rinsed and drained

2 medium zucchini

4 stalks celery

1 medium onion

½ cup salsa

3 cups broth (vegetable or chicken, I prefer low-sodium)

2 cloves garlic, minced

½ teaspoon chili powder (or more to taste)

½ teaspoon salt

½ teaspoon ground black pepper

2 teaspoon ground cumin

1 tablespoon olive oil

INSTRUCTIONS

Spray a large crockpot with olive oil or cooking spray.

Chop onion, celery, and zucchini into bite-sized pieces.

Add all ingredients to crockpot, and stir.

Cook on high for 1 hour, then on low for about 6 hours or until ready to serve.

Serve topped with avocado, parmesan cheese, or Greek yogurt (a great substitute for sour cream!).

~ Recipe: Sizzlin' Southwestern Spaghetti Squash ~

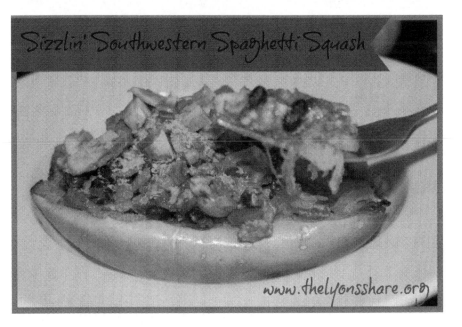

Sizzlin' Southwestern Spaghetti Squash is as fun to eat as it is to say. Each serving is a large "boat" made of half of a spaghetti squash, filled with flavorful and delicious toppings. If you choose, feel free to use ground turkey, chicken, or lean ground beef instead of the crumbled tempeh.

Makes 2 servings. Each serving will contain 381 calories, 10g fat, 50g carbs, and 20g protein.

INGREDIENTS

1 medium-sized spaghetti squash

½ onion (white or yellow)

10 cherry tomatoes

2 tsp. cumin, divided

1 tsp. garlic powder, divided

½ block (about 150g) tempeh

⅔ cup black beans, drained and rinsed

4 Tbsp. salsa

2 tsp. fire-roasted chiles

⅓ avocado

4 Tbsp. nutritional yeast or parmesan cheese

INSTRUCTIONS

Pre-heat oven to 400 degrees.

Poke a few holes in your spaghetti squash so air can escape and it doesn't explode when heated. Microwave for 3 minutes to soften. When squash is cool enough to handle, slice lengthwise, scoop out seeds and stringy flesh, and place open-side down on a foil-lined baking pan sprayed with cooking spray. Bake 30 minutes.

Meanwhile, dice onion and slice tomatoes into halves or quarters. Spray a pan with cooking spray or olive oil, and add onion, 1 tsp. cumin, and 1/2 tsp. garlic powder. Sauté until beginning to soften. Add tomatoes and sauté an additional 2-3 minutes.

After 30 minutes, remove your spaghetti squash and flip the halves over (so the inside faces up). Sprinkle with the remainder of your cumin and garlic powder, and return to oven for 10-15 more minutes, or until edges are starting to brown.

Add crumbled tempeh to onion and tomatoes. (You can crumble it with your hands, until it looks approximately like ground beef or turkey). Add rinsed and drained black beans and green chiles, and sauté an additional 5 minutes.

Add salsa to pan and stir until heated through.

Place one half of spaghetti squash into a bowl, and spoon in half of the filling. Top with half of the chopped avocado and 2 tablespoons of nutritional yeast or parmesan cheese.

~ Recipe: Grab-and-Go Egg Muffins ~

For those who always are running out of the house 5 minutes late in the morning, but still want a nutritious and tasty breakfast, Grab-and-Go Egg Muffins can be easily reheated from the refrigerator or freezer.

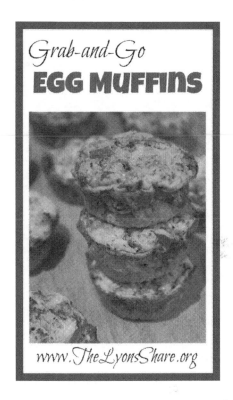

Makes 12 muffins. Each muffin will contain 54 calories, 1.5g fat, 4.5g carbs, and 5.5g protein.

I generally eat 3 muffins, alongside cherry tomatoes, avocado slices, and a piece of fruit.

INGREDIENTS

9 eggs (or substitute 1.5 cups of liquid egg whites)

12 Tbsp. cooked quinoa

1 cup broccoli

1 cup cauliflower

1 medium red pepper

1 tsp. dried basil

½ tsp. salt

½ tsp. ground black pepper

Optional: ¼ - ½ cup salsa

INSTRUCTIONS

Preheat oven to 350 degrees.

Spray muffin tin (12 cups) with olive oil or cooking spray.

Place 1 Tbsp. of cooked quinoa into each tin.

Lightly steam all vegetables (in microwave or steamer), and finely chop. Evenly distribute vegetables into muffin tins, on top of quinoa.

Beat eggs and egg substitute (or egg whites) with spices and salsa, if using.

Spoon egg mixture into muffin tins, on top of quinoa and vegetables.

Bake for 15-18 minutes, or until tops are just beginning to brown.

Note: Feel free to substitute any vegetables you choose. For more flavor, experiment with a variety of spices and herbs.

~ Recipe: Just Like Mom's Chunky Mashed Cauliflower ~

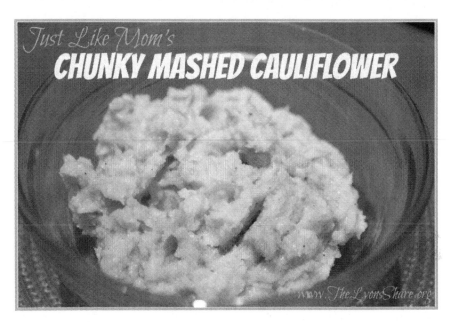

Cheesy, warm, and comforting, this Chunky Mashed Cauliflower is a great way to disguise veggies, even for picky kids!

Makes 2 servings. Each serving will contain 116 calories, 1g fat, 22g carbs, and 6g protein.

INGREDIENTS

2 cups packed, chopped cauliflower

1 large parsnip (about 150g)

2 Tbsp. nutritional yeast or parmesan cheese

¼ cup skim milk, or unsweetened plain milk substitute

¼ tsp. each of salt and pepper, or to taste

INSTRUCTIONS

Roughly chop cauliflower and parsnip, and place in large, covered, microwave-safe bowl (or place in steamer).

Microwave for 8 minutes, or until vegetables are soft.

Place all ingredients in a blender, and puree. I prefer my mashed cauliflower with a few chunks, but feel free to puree until silky smooth if you like it that way!

~ Recipe: Summer RefreshMINT Smoothie ~

A great introduction to green smoothies, this smoothie has a mint-flavor that makes its green color more appealing to skeptics. Enjoy this refreshing summery smoothie at any time of year – just imagine you're on a tropical beach!

Makes 1 large smoothie. Each smoothie contains 225 calories, 6.5g fat, 33g carbs, and 17g protein.

INGREDIENTS

1 scoop vanilla flavored protein powder (I like Juice Plus+ Complete Protein for this smoothie; purchase at MeganLyons.JuicePlus.com)

½ cup cucumber

2 cups romaine lettuce

½ cup unsweetened vanilla almond milk (or other unsweetened milk or milk substitute)

1/6 medium avocado

½ cup frozen pineapple

1 cup water

3-4 sprigs of fresh mint leaves

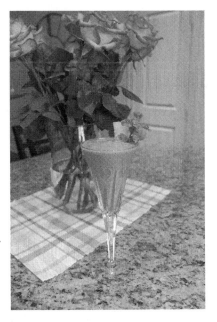

INSTRUCTIONS

Add all ingredients to high-powered blender, and blend until smooth.

Enjoy!

CHAPTER FOUR

TOO SWEET TO BE TRUE

*I*magine stirring a teaspoon of sugar into your coffee or tea. Now imagine doing that 14,021 times over the course of the year, or 39.4 times a day. It may seem excessive, but that is the amount of added sugar the average American consumed in 2000, according to the USDA.[30] The 152.4 pounds of added sugar we consume each year not only lead us to crave more and more sugar, but also are a major reason that our waistlines are increasing and our health is eroding.

Sugar is being added to nearly all packaged food, from sauces and dressings, to yogurt and cereal bars, to juices and sodas. Two table-spoons of KC Masterpiece Original barbecue sauce contain a full three teaspoons of sugar, as does a ½-cup serving of Newman's Own Organic Tomato & Basil Sauce. Even healthier sounding products often contain large quantities of sugar – a ¾-cup serving of Kellogg's Cracklin' Oat Bran contains 3.5 teaspoons of sugar (14 grams)[31] ... and very few people eat only ¾ cup!

It's nearly impossible – and unnecessary – to avoid sugar altogether. However, limiting our consumption of *added* sugar – while difficult – is one of the most important steps we can take toward maintaining a healthy weight, balanced energy levels, and overall optimal health.

Overview: Sugar and Its Impact on Our Health

What do we mean when we say "sugar," anyway? From a science perspective, "sugar" is a category that refers to a group of carbohydrates, from simple sugars like sucrose (table sugar) to more complex sugars (like starch). There are so many types of sugar that it can be hard to identify them or tell them apart (in fact, nearly 100 approved names for sugar, syrups, and other sweeteners appear on our food labels). However, you can generally tell if something is a sugar if it ends in "-ose."

Glucose, one of the simplest forms of sugar, provides the cells of the human body with a source of energy, and is the preferred source of fuel for the brain, nervous system, and red blood cells. Given that, you might expect that consuming lots of sugar would lead to increased energy, brain function, and improved overall health, but that could hardly be further from the truth.

In fact, as the average consumption of sugar has skyrocketed, our health overall has deteriorated, and sugar is at least partly to blame. Excess sugar, and especially excess added sugar, has been linked to numerous chronic diseases, and most scientific and governmental organizations now recommend significant decreases in consumption.

Recently, the World Health Organization published a "strong" recommendation to reduce consumption of added sugars. The report clearly stated that when added sugars comprise 10 percent or more of the diet, there is higher risk for weight gain, childhood obesity, and dental cavities. In countries where added sugar consumption totaled less than 5 percent of total calorie intake, children fared even better than when the sugar intake comprised 10 percent of the diet.[32]

That is a huge finding! Childhood obesity has more than doubled in children (and quadrupled in adolescents) over the past 30 years.[33] and this is directly correlated to the increase in sugar. If we want to gain control of the childhood obesity problem, we're going to have to start limiting added sugar.

The weight problem doesn't stop with children. Added sugar is contributing to our weight problems, and reducing it is one of the most surefire ways to lose weight.

Let's do some math. 16 percent of the average American's daily calorie intake comes from added sugar.[34] With an average of 2,270 calories a day, we are getting 363 calories a day from added sugar, or 132,568 calories per year. If we could reduce that by just a third, we'd save 44,189 calories per year, which equates to *12.6 pounds* of body weight per year. So if you are trying to lose weight, cutting back on added sugar is an easy way to do so.

Added sugar also increases the risk of Type 2 diabetes. The development of Type 2 diabetes long has been linked to obesity, and because many foods with added sugar are high in calories, added sugar has been linked to diabetes.

New research shows that the connection goes beyond simple weight gain. Researchers at UC San Francisco showed that increased sugar in a given population's food supply was linked to higher Type 2 diabetes rates, even when controlling for factors like obesity, physical activity, other types of calories, and other economic and social factors.[35] So it's not just that sugar leads to weight gain, which leads to higher risk of diabetes; it's the actual sugar itself that may increase our risk for Type 2 diabetes!

The following chart, from "The Relationship of Sugar to Population-Level Diabetes Prevalence: An Econometric Analysis of Repeated Cross-Sectional Data" by Basu, Yoffee, Hills, & Lustig, shows a direct correlation between the increase in sugar availability and the prevalence of diabetes. Simply put, when we make sugar more available, diabetes prevalence increases, and when we reduce the availability of sugar, diabetes incidence falls.

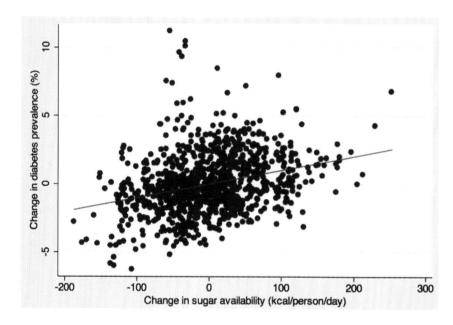

If weight gain and diabetes weren't enough to convince you that sugar is significantly undermining our health, the health risks of eating a diet high in sugar go even further. A 2014 study in the *Journal of the American Medical Association* found that those who consumed 25 percent of their daily calories from sugar were more than twice as likely to die from heart disease as those whose sugar intake was less than 10 percent of total calorie intake.[36]

A groundbreaking 2007 study in the *American Journal of Clinical Nutrition* concluded that increased sugar consumption contributed to or caused the increased prevalence of hypertension, obesity, diabetes, kidney disease, cardiovascular disease, and metabolic syndrome.[37] Yet again, we see direct data showing that as sugar consumption increases, obesity and disease increase right alongside it.

Sugar can also block hormone receptors, making those who consume it in excess less responsive to insulin (and more susceptible to blood sugar swings or feelings of instability). It can weaken bone and muscle, impair mood and memory, cause arthritis and premature aging, and even make cancer and infection more likely.[38] A process called glycation, through which sugar makes cells and tissues stiff, can cause red blood cells to become bloated and ultimately impair circulation. Some research links increased consumption of sugar to birth defects, dementia, and abnormally high cholesterol.

An abundance of added sugar not only contributes to Type 2 diabetes, obesity, and insulin resistance, it also reduces your immune system's function, and can contribute to high cholesterol (especially high triglycerides), arthritis, heart disease, depression, osteoporosis, and more. Basically, sugar isn't doing us any favors, and is significantly detracting from our overall health. A teaspoon of sugar here or a small piece of candy there is certainly not going to kill you, but it's very rare that we're limiting ourselves to small amounts. Sugar is so prevalent in our food supply, and so addictive, that most of us consume far more than we even realize.

More Addictive than Cocaine: The Addictive Properties of Sugar

Given the numerous health risks associated with sugar, it may seem obvious that any well-educated person would reduce consumption immediately. Yet, intake of sugar continues to skyrocket! Unfortunately, the amount of available sugar in our food supply is increasing steadily, and humans are hard-wired to consume it. The National Academy of Sciences cites a "biological drive" to eat sugar for survival.[39] Our brains have natural reward systems that release dopamine and other "feel-good chemicals" that make us want to do the things that are necessary for human survival. This is part of the reason why mothers feel good when they take care of their kids, and why eating and having sex make us feel good – we need to do them to ensure that the human species lives on. Hundreds of years ago, when there wasn't much sugar available, our ancestors were encouraged to eat sugar by their natural reward systems, since sugar would help them hold onto weight and avoid starvation.

Today, many of us are fortunate to not wonder where our next meal will come from, and there is no shortage of calories in most of our homes. Cultural patterns like birthday celebrations and Halloween candy fests, mass media advertisements, and other stresses of modern life have only increased the emphasis we put on sugar, and its constant presence in our lives. We are constantly bombarded with images of sugar; we are constantly offered sugar-containing treats; and we are constantly thinking about sugar ... all of which fuels the sugar craze to the level of an addiction.

A study published in 2007 took this biological drive even further, showing that the addictive potential of sugar is even higher than that of cocaine.[40] The researchers had laboratory rats choose between sweetened water and an IV of cocaine, and 94 percent of the rats chose the sweet taste. Even those that were already "hooked" on cocaine chose the sweet water! This goes to show that the term "sugar addiction" is more accurate than most of us know: Sugar truly is an addiction, and the vast majority of Americans today are addicts. "Bet you can't eat just one" and "once you pop, you can't stop" are not only catchy slogans, they are truths of the modern American: We're consuming too much sugar, and we truly can't stop.

In fact, the modern food supply makes things far worse. We now get sweetness not only from whole fruit, but from concentrated sweeteners like corn syrup and artificial sweeteners, which are often thousands of times sweeter than pure sugar. As manufacturers pour more and more sweeteners into food products, and as access to these processed food products becomes more and more convenient, we consume more sugar-filled "products" and less whole food. The average American now consumes about 60 percent of his calories from processed food.[41] and 71 percent of packaged food products sold in supermarkets contain added sugar![42]

Because humans evolved without access to the intense sweetness provided by the artificial ingredients and chemically-refined food products of today, today's human brains react to this intense sweetness by giving an equally intense reward in the form of a dopamine release. This reward is thought to be so satisfying that it has the "potential to override self-control mechanisms."[43] The addictive potential of sugar, then, makes it very difficult for a modern consumer, who has been exposed to heavily refined foods and added sugars, to stop consuming so much.

Added Sugar vs. Natural Sugar

You may have noticed that many of the research studies mentioned so far talk about *added* sugar (which is the sugar added to foods by manufacturers, cooks, or consumers, and also includes sugars in honey, syrups, juices, and juice concentrates). From a health perspective, this is different from naturally occurring sugar (such as the sugar in fruits, vegetables, and dairy products). Some health experts claim that we need to limit added sugar only, while others recommend limiting total sugars (including naturally-occurring and added). Let's explore both sides.

The World Health Organization states that "no reported evidence" links the consumption of intrinsic (naturally occurring) sugars to adverse health effects.[44] Because most naturally occurring sugar is packaged together with fiber, phytonutrients, and antioxidants (such as in the case of fruit or starchy vegetables), the human body is better able to process naturally occurring sugar. Our bodies recognize naturally occurring sugar as food, and can use it appropriately, so it is less likely to cause health issues.

Still, this is not a license to forget about your vegetables and consume an abundance of fruit day in and day out. Naturally occurring complex carbohydrates (such as starchy vegetables and fruits) take more time to be absorbed into the bloodstream, but they also stay in the bloodstream longer, giving our blood sugar a rise for a longer period of time. If you're exercising or expending energy, this is a good thing, but if you're sedentary, you may not need as much fruit or starch as you think you do. Too much fructose (the type of sugar found in fruit) may even encourage the liver to enter fat-storage mode, and contribute to conditions like fatty liver. This is bad news for Durianrider and Freelee, two YouTube stars who claim to eat 30-51 bananas a day each! (Without meaning to offend them, I believe this is proof that people will do anything to make a splash, and that fad diets continue to get more and more extreme!)

In my opinion, the answer lies somewhere in between these two extremes. While I believe the majority of the damage is caused by *added* sugar, I also encourage clients to use the naturally occurring sugars in fruits as sweet treats, and to choose nutrient-dense vegetables for the majority of their carbohydrate intake. In my experience, limiting added sugar as much as possible, and keeping fruit to a few servings a day contributes to a more stable blood sugar, fewer sweet cravings, and reduced overall calorie intake.

Here's my bottom line: Eat as many non-starchy vegetables as you'd like, and sprinkle in starchy vegetables and fruits as complements. Limit the *added* sugar as much as possible, and you'll be on your way to great health!

High Fructose Corn Syrup: The Root of All of Our Problems?

Now you know that naturally occurring sugar is a whole lot better than added sugar, but are there types of added sugar that are better than others? Many clients come to me shunning chemical-sounding sweeteners like high fructose corn syrup, but using agave nectar or coconut palm sugar liberally. Is this a good idea?

The blame for the increase in added sugar consumption often is placed on the increased usage of high fructose corn syrup, a sweet syrup used by manufacturers to enhance the sweetness of refined foods at low cost. Some believe that the high fructose-to-glucose ratio in high-fructose corn syrup may make the body more likely to store it as fat, and thus contribute to excess weight gain. But there hasn't been any conclusive research showing this.

In a similar vein, the popularity of agave nectar has skyrocketed over the past decade, after the media touted it as a "healthier" alternative to traditional sweeteners like sugar or honey, since it comes from a plant. Unfortunately, there's no "free lunch" when it comes to nutrition, and there's just as much sugar in agave nectar as there is in honey or similar sweeteners (and sometimes even more calories). While many say it is healthier because it has a lower glycemic index (meaning that it spikes your blood sugar less dramatically than an alternative), it also has a higher concentration of fructose, which may lead to health issues like diabetes or fatty liver.

We could go on and on, but suffice it to say that there is no form of added sugar that is *good* for you. The closest to an ideal are honey and real maple syrup, which are both rich in vitamins and minerals, so at least you're getting some benefit with your sugar. Even with honey and maple syrup, though, an abundance of sugar is not doing your health any favors.

It's OK to include a little bit of sweetener every once in a while, but nearly everyone would feel better and improve their health if their added sugar consumption were reduced.

Sugar Substitutes: A Free Pass?

If added sugar of all kinds is harmful to health, then, should you make the switch to artificial sweeteners? The pink, blue, and yellow packets (Sweet & Low, Equal, and Splenda, respectively) can be found almost everywhere, and many people automatically assume that they are a healthier option than the regular sugar packets.

When artificial sweeteners (such as aspartame, acesulfame potassium, saccharin, and sucralose) first began gaining popularity, research showing they may increase the risk of cancer scared many people away.[45] There are also studies, though, that show no correlation at all, and even some that show that substituting artificial sweeteners for sugar may *reduce* the risk of cancer.[46] The FDA refutes the connection between artificial sweeteners and cancer, saying that "based on the available scientific evidence, the agency has concluded that the high-intensity sweeteners approved by the FDA are safe for the general population."[47]

The bottom line is that we don't know enough to say whether or not artificial sweeteners are linked to cancer. We need more research before we can definitively say either way. But, don't go reaching for your pink packet yet!

In addition to cancer, artificial sweeteners raise several other health concerns. Research shows that those who consume more artificially sweetened beverages (like diet sodas) have higher incidence of

Type 2 diabetes.[48] Artificial sweeteners often cause gastrointestinal distress (like bloating, gas, and diarrhea). In fact, many of my clients report that they never even realized they were so bloated, until they reduced their intake of artificial sweeteners and noticed their waistline shrinking or didn't have the uncomfortable "puffy" feeling they assumed was just "normal!"

What's more, we can't ignore that the substances in the pink, blue, and yellow packets are chemicalized, highly unnatural products that our bodies don't recognize as food. Did you know that Splenda (sucralose) is made by adding three chlorine molecules (yes, the stuff we put in our swimming pools!) to one sugar molecule? The chlorine molecules are added so the body won't recognize the sugar molecule, and can't absorb the calories from the sugar. But the act of putting a chemical into your body to trick it seems (and is) unnatural, and there are always consequences to tricking your body.

Still, you might think that artificial sweeteners are worth the risk, if they'll help you lose weight. Not so fast! The impact of artificial sweeteners on weight maintenance is unclear: Some studies show they are helpful in reducing weight, while others show they may even contribute to weight gain by limiting the body's ability to gauge how many calories have been consumed.[49] In myself and in many of my clients, an increase in artificial sweeteners leads to more sugar cravings throughout the day, so the calorie-free artificial sweetener packet still leads to an increase in overall calories consumed.

The bottom line is that we don't know enough to say that artificial sweeteners are either definitively harmful, or definitively safe, so I recommend limiting or avoiding them until the science advances.

Your best bet is to reduce both added sugar and artificial sweeteners, but going cold turkey may be too difficult. If you really want to limit your calorie intake by avoiding added sugar, but want to stay away from the risks associated with artificial sweeteners, stevia may be a good stepping-stone. Stevia is derived from a plant, so it's far more natural than the chemicalized products in the pink, blue, and yellow packets. It is still calorie-free, and it is 200 times sweeter than sugar, so you need to use far less. There is some research showing potential health benefits of stevia (like lowering blood pressure), but also some showing that stevia may make you crave more sweet treats, just as artificial sweeteners do. So, I don't recommend going overboard on stevia, but I do suggest it as a healthy upgrade from artificial sweeteners, and as a way to transition to using no sweetener at all (or, at least, very little sweetener).

How to start Reducing Your Sugar Intake: Choosing an Approach

If you've gotten this far through the chapter, you are (hopefully) motivated to begin reducing your sugar intake. It sounds like a good idea ... you know it's good for your long-term health ... it's bound to make you feel better. But it's still *very* overwhelming to start. I understand that, and I've been there. Sugar is so pervasive in our food supply, and – let's face it – so tasty, that it's hard to know where to start.

The American Heart Association recommends keeping added sugar intake to 6 teaspoons (or 24 grams, or about 100 calories) for women, and 9 teaspoons (or 36 grams, or about 150 calories) for men each day.[50] This is about 25 percent of what the average American is actually taking in, and I think it's a great goal to strive for. Of course, I'd love it if added sugar intake were nearly zero, but I know how difficult that is in our busy world. Now that we know what we're striving to achieve, let's get down to business.

There are two major schools of thought on how to successfully reduce sugar intake. The first, made popular by cleanses and overly restrictive "miracle diets," is to go cold turkey. One benefit of going cold turkey is that there's no room for false interpretation (meaning you can't say "well, this cookie is half the size of the cookie I usually get, and look, it has oatmeal in it ... so it *must* be healthy!"). For those who thrive on following directions, and who tend to have a "black and white" mentality, going cold turkey can be appealing. After all, there's a "can" and a "cannot" list, and there's no guesswork or judgment involved. You don't have to think; you just follow the directions.

As we've learned, sugar is addictive, so by taking it out altogether, we're less likely to fall into the trap of having just one bite ... then wanting more and more. It's also a quicker process and, because sugar is so harmful to our health, breaking from the addiction sooner is a good thing.

Despite the benefits of going cold turkey, though, I still don't recommend it. Primarily, because it's just too hard for most people, and sets them up for failure, rebound bingeing, or self-deprecation. In general, when someone who is consuming a large amount of sugar on a regular basis tries to give it up completely, he or she can stick with it for a day or two. Some may succeed for a week, and some may not even last a few hours. Inevitably, though, a bit of sugar creeps in (consciously or unconsciously), and we assume that we have "blown it." Because of this black-and-white mentality, we often end up eating even more sugar than we otherwise would have. For the same reason that we go back for a *third* plate at Thanksgiving when we're already stuffed, or that we order the triple layer chocolate cake *after* we've enjoyed an appetizer, salad, and indulgent main course, we often "throw in the towel" once we've strayed from our plan.

If this cycle of committing to perfection then bingeing continues, we deepen our addiction, making it harder and harder to eventually give up sugar. It's possible to run into blood sugar stability issues, and probable that the person will feel defeated and eventually give up on trying to eliminate sugar.

Withdrawal symptoms also are far greater when giving up sugar cold turkey. Remember, sugar is as addictive, or more addictive, than many drugs, so your body will make it difficult for you to quit it by presenting you with headaches, nausea, intense cravings, shakiness, fatigue, and mild depression. These are unpleasant and mostly avoidable by tapering off more slowly.

For all of these reasons, I prefer to remove sugar gradually. While tapering sugar from your diet takes more time and allows more room for judgment, I have seen time and again that it is the approach that leads to more long-term success. A gradual process allows a person to actually change her habits, rather than following a "diet plan" that inevitably ends and invites back old behaviors.

Withdrawal symptoms are reduced with a gradual approach, and there is more time to replace sugar-laden habits and behaviors with new, healthier behaviors. Once you transition to a lower sugar lifestyle, it may even become hard to remember the days of pastry breakfasts and vending machine candy bar runs!

As you go through the gradual approach, you may find yourself missing some of the sugary foods you used to consume regularly. At first, the approach may feel restrictive or "unfair" ... you may find yourself thinking things like, "why can everyone else consume all the Twinkies and sugary cereal they want, without an impact on their health?" The truth, though, is that the sugar *is* negatively impacting them, and that the health of our nation is in grave danger. Plus, it's really of no use comparing yourself to others. You know that you are making the decision to reduce your own sugar intake for your own health, and that's all that matters.

You may be thinking "but I *really* like ____!" I understand ... sugar *does* taste good. However, by committing to reducing the sugar from your diet right now, you are *not* saying that you'll never choose to have a cookie or a piece of Halloween candy again. I think that is unrealistic for most people, and not an approach I recommend or follow myself. If you commit to a few weeks of gradually reducing your sugar, though, I can almost guarantee that you'll feel the impact so strongly that you won't want to go back to eating as much sugar as you're used to eating. As strange as it sounds, once you wean yourself off the constant sugar high that most of us are riding, the sugar will actually be *less* appealing when you do have it.

You may have eaten tons of sugar for years, and felt fine, but it *will* catch up to you sooner or later if you don't reverse the practice. So, commit now to gradually reducing the sugar in your diet!

The Gradual Approach: Removing Obvious Sources of Sugar

I recommend starting with the obvious sources of sugar first (then attacking my top 15 sources of hidden sugar once you've weaned yourself off of the obvious sources). To start, think about the past 48 hours. Have you poured sugar in your coffee? Eaten donuts for breakfast or brownies after dinner? Are you a regular soda consumer? The area that stands out most to you is likely the most glaring offender, and is the best area to attack first.

I suggest taking away one source of added sugar each week. For example, you may start by replacing soda with water this week, and focus on it every day until it slowly becomes a habit. After a week, or once you feel comfortable with the replacement, then take out your afternoon cookie, or your morning donut. Going one by one feels less overwhelming, and will allow you time to figure out substitutes for the things you consume most frequently.

Today, the average American gets 46 percent of her added sugar from sugar-sweetened soft drinks.[51] There are 65 grams of sugar (over 16 teaspoons!) in a 32-ounce fast-food cup of soda, and cup sizes seem to be ever-expanding. So, if you regularly consume soda, this is a great place to start. Try swapping out one soda a day for tea (black, green, or herbal all have great health benefits), no-sugar-added sparkling water, or water infused with fresh fruit. Once you have successfully traded one soda a day, trade another one every week until you have weaned yourself off of soda altogether.

If your office has candy bowls or jars in plain sight, chances are you're consuming more candy than you realize on a daily basis. Just 10 M&Ms on your way back from the restroom adds up to 111 grams of sugar, or 28 teaspoons, per week (if you go to the restroom 5 times a day and work 5 days a week). Start with just one day, and commit to avoiding the candy jar each time you pass it. If you make it through the whole day, put a star on your calendar or use another congratulatory method to keep track of your success. Slowly, you can break yourself of the habit!

If you add sugar into your coffee, cereal, fruit, or anything else, you'll want to cut back on this next. My clients often tell me, "I only use a teaspoon, which only has 16 calories!" This is true, but if you drink 2 cups of coffee a day, you're adding 11,680 calories per year, or about 3.3 pounds of extra body weight. Far more important than the weight, though, is the continuous spike in your blood sugar. As you get in the habit of "stoking the fire" with added sugar, your body becomes less and less sensitive to the impact of insulin, and you can eventually set yourself up for longer term health consequences.

Next, consider any cookies, cake, pastries, ice cream, donuts, or other sweet treats you eat regularly. When you eat these things, how do you feel an hour later? My guess is that you are experiencing a sugar crash, likely resulting in an energy slump (just like kids who are bouncing off the walls on a sugar high, then end up passed out in bed when the high wears off). If you're not experiencing an energy slump, ask yourself if you're constantly stoking the fire with more sugar throughout the day. When my clients report that they felt "snacky" all day, or just couldn't seem to feel satisfied, they often have started their day with a sugary option, like a pastry or a bowl of sugary cereal. When we reduce the sugar in their breakfasts, they often are amazed by how their entire day seems more nutritionally balanced, and by how their cravings are dramatically reduced. So, if you consume any of these regularly, the next step is to reduce them.

If you're thinking, "I only consume cookies on special occasions," or something similar to that, I encourage you to think about what is truly a special occasion. For so many people, sweets are brought into the workplace nearly every day, as they celebrate a coworker's birthday, a holiday, or a success at work. If these are truly special occasions, I have no problem with indulging in a treat every once in a while. However, if you think your "special occasions" are adding up to a daily occurrence, it may be time to reassess your definition.

If you're worried about how your birthday or Christmas Day will ever be the same without your special sweet treat, remind yourself that this is not forever. For now, focus on enjoying the celebration of the holiday – being with family, participating in traditions, and taking time away from your regular routine. I'll venture to guess that once you realize how great you feel on a reduced sugar diet, and once you learn to enjoy holidays for what they are (rather than focusing on the food), you're less likely to want to overdose on sugar, even on special occasions. But I'll let you figure this out for yourself. For now, don't get bogged down in the "forever" mentality; just commit to going step-by-step, week-by-week to reduce the obvious sugar offenders in your diet.

Hidden Sugars: The Top 15 Sources

Once you've successfully reduced your intake of the obvious sources of sugar, it's time to move on to the hidden sources of sugar. You may be surprised by how some of these healthy-sounding foods pack in just as much sugar as the obvious offenders from the previous section. Unfortunately, as food manufacturers attempt to make their products taste great at low cost, they have become adept at adding sweeteners to products that were never traditionally sweet. Often, products labeled "low fat" or "fat free" have far more sugar than their "regular" counterparts, so beware of misleading health claims.

Just as you did with the obvious sources of sugar, I recommend going one-at-a-time for the hidden sugar categories. Making gradual changes is far more sustainable and less overwhelming, so you're more likely to stick to your new habits for the long run. Which of these items do you consume regularly? Choose one, replace it with a healthier alternative for a week, and move on to the next. Gradually, you'll reduce a great deal of added sugar, and begin feeling better and better!

Here are my top 15 sources of added sugar, along with tips on how to upgrade or replace them:

1. **SPAGHETTI SAUCE:** It might be one of the last places you'd expect to find added sugar, but most pre-prepared spaghetti sauce is loaded with it. A ½-cup serving of Prego Tomato, Onion, & Garlic sauce has 12 grams of sugar, or 3 teaspoons, and most of it is added sugar ("sugar" falls right after "dehydrated onions" on the ingredient list). Most people use double or triple the serving size, which means they could easily have

the same amount of sugar as a can of Coke ... right on top of their pasta! Replace it with plain canned tomato sauce with some Italian seasoning stirred in (a ½-cup has 4 grams of naturally occurring sugar), or simply sauté some fresh tomatoes, onions, garlic, basil, and oregano in olive oil.

2. **BARBECUE SAUCE:** Two tablespoons of KC Masterpiece Original barbecue sauce contain a full three teaspoons of sugar. I recall my family making barbecued chicken with about a half a bottle of barbecue sauce (a whopping 51 teaspoons of sugar, split among our 4-person family), so I think it's safe to say that it can quickly add up. To upgrade your barbecue sauce, try marinating chicken in olive oil, lemon juice, and herbs. Even if you "must" spread a thin layer of barbecue sauce on after cooking, you're still reducing your intake dramatically. If you want to make your own barbecue sauce, just Google "low sugar barbecue sauce recipe," and you'll come up with several options.

3. **KETCHUP:** I love ketchup, and remember fondly squeezing nearly a full ketchup packet (3 grams of sugar!) onto each French fry in my childhood days. The third ingredient in Heinz ketchup is high fructose corn syrup, and the fourth is corn syrup – just picture a ketchup bottle a quarter-full of sugar, and that's exactly what you're putting on your burger! I recommend swapping for tomato slices or salsa, which give a lot of flavor with low calories and no added sugar. If you prefer to make an added-sugar-free ketchup, there are also several recipes available online.

4. **SALAD DRESSING:** By now, you're probably noticing a trend: Many sauces tend to be sugar-laden. Salad dressings are no exception, and the ones labeled "fat-free" are often the worst culprits, since food manufacturers have to enhance the taste

with something (added sugar!) after removing the fat. Two tablespoons of Kraft Fat-Free Raspberry Vinaigrette dressing have 9 grams of sugar. In fact, the dressing contains more sugar than vinegar, oil, raspberry, or anything else aside from water! To upgrade your dressing, look for dressings with 2 grams or less per serving. I recommend using olive oil and balsamic vinegar or lemon juice. I often enjoy dressing a salad simply with avocado oil and salt, or sometimes use salsa and avocado for a Mexican-inspired salad. Be creative, but stay away from the sugary prepared options when you can.

5. **YOGURT:** You may think that you're making the healthier choice by opting for yogurt at breakfast, but if you're reaching for a version laden with added sugars, you may be wrong. Yogurt is one of the top places food manufacturers hide added sugar – a 6-ounce container of Yoplait Strawberry has 25 grams of sugar (more than 6 teaspoons!), and Kraft Breyers Smooth & Creamy Lowfat Strawberry Yogurt has a whopping 39 grams (nearly 10 teaspoons). I'm sure you can't imagine pouring 10 teaspoons of sugar directly into your mouth, so it's best to shy away from these versions. Any yogurt will have *some* sugar, because milk products contain lactose, a naturally-occurring sugar. A plain 6-ounce serving of Fage 0 percent Greek yogurt contains 7 grams, for example. Remember to check the ingredient list to see if sugar (or any of its many other names, such as corn syrup, high fructose corn syrup, maltose, dextrose, fructose, corn syrup, cane syrup, maple syrup, or molasses) are high in the ranking. In general, I recommend staying away from any yogurt with more than 15 grams of sugar per serving. It is helpful to choose plain varieties (rather than fruit flavored varieties), and add your own flavoring with berries, other chopped fruit, canned pumpkin and cinnamon, or cocoa powder and stevia

for a chocolatey treat. Even adding a small drizzle of honey or maple syrup will give you far less added sugar than the pre-sweetened varieties.

6. **MUFFINS**: Another innocent-sounding culprit, the muffin might be one of the sneakiest sources of added sugar there is. Even the healthier-sounding muffins at Starbucks contain up to 34 grams (they have recently redone their menu, as previous versions had up to 57 grams of sugar each!), and it's not just Starbucks. The Cinnamon Crumb muffin at Corner Bakery has 50 grams; the Coffee Cake muffin at Dunkin' Donuts has 51 grams (in fact, you could have 5 Bavarian Cream donuts for less sugar!). The best upgrade for lower-sugar muffins is to make your own. See my recipe for Zucchini Apple Breakfast Muffins at the end of this chapter, or look for other recipes, clocking in at no more than 10 grams of sugar each (ideally from naturally occurring sources).

7. **ENERGY BARS, PROTEIN BARS, GRANOLA BARS**: If I had a dollar for every time a client told me they ate an energy bar instead of an apple, thinking they were making a healthy decision, I would be a happy camper. Not only do most energy bars contain preservatives, artificial sweeteners, and more chemical-sounding ingredients than you can imagine, but they often contain high amounts of added sugar. A Clif bar – often touted as a healthy snack – contains 24 grams of sugar. The first ingredient (even before oats!) is brown rice syrup, a source of added sugar. The "Performance Energy" PowerBar contains 28 grams of sugar, and the first ingredient is a combination of various types of sugars. Of course, this is far less harmful if you're in the act of running a marathon or a multi-hour bike ride, but for the average person picking up a bar in the checkout aisle of the supermarket, the sugar is doing more harm than good. To upgrade your bars, look for bars that have only naturally occurring sugar (Larabars, for

example, are fairly high in total sugar, at 18 grams each, but the sugar comes from fruit only, rather than added sugar). Lower sugar, higher protein bars are also available, and are great options for many people, but the "best" bar really varies by person. Depending on the clients' goals, the sensitivity of their stomachs, their dietary restrictions, and their preferences, there are a wide range of bars I frequently recommend. Regardless, I recommend choosing one with minimal added sugar, at least 3 grams of fiber, and at least 5 grams of protein and/or healthy fat.

8. **GRANOLA:** Once touted as the go-to option for health-conscious people, one cup of granola can come out to over 600 calories – before adding milk or toppings – because of all the added sugar. To upgrade your morning bowl, always check the serving sizes of granola, which are often ¼ to ⅓ cup (a small fraction of the size of a normal cereal bowl), and limit yourself to a single serving. Look for varieties that include naturally occurring sweeteners rather than adding in simple sugar. Better yet, make your own granola at home, so you can limit the amount of sweetener you add.

9. **BREAKFAST CEREAL:** As mentioned earlier in the chapter, starting your day with a high dosage of added sugar sets you up for more cravings throughout the day, and leads to general blood sugar instability. What a shame, then, that so many of the foods we feed our children first thing in the morning contain so much added sugar! There are the obvious sources, like Kellogg's Froot Loops, which clock in at 13 grams per serving and contain more sugar than anything else, and Kellogg's Honey Smacks (branded initially as "Sugar Smacks"), which are over 50 percent sugar by weight. And it's not just the indulgent-sounding varieties that are sugar bombs. Even healthier sounding products often contain large quantities of sugar – a 1-cup serving

of Post Raisin Bran contains 19 grams of sugar (nearly 5 teaspoons), and a ¾-cup serving of Kellogg's Cracklin' Oat Bran contains 14 grams. To upgrade your cereal, first watch your portion sizes. It can be helpful to measure out a correct portion at least a few times, so you learn to eyeball the appropriate size. Second, choose a healthier cereal. I recommend looking for a cereal with less than 8 grams of sugar per serving, at least 3 grams of fiber, and at least 3 grams of protein or healthy fat. There are some available cereals that contain just one ingredient, the grain itself (for example, puffed millet or puffed kamut). I also recommend that clients add in a tablespoon of chia seeds or slivered almonds to their cereal bowl, to provide a bit of extra healthy fat that will slow the blood sugar spike, and some optional blueberries, to provide a good dose of micronutrients to start the day.

10. **DRIED FRUIT:** If dried fruit seems too delicious to be healthy, unfortunately, it probably is. Not only do most food manufacturers add in significant amounts of sugar to sweeten the dried fruit, but the process of drying removes water, which concentrates even the naturally-occurring sugar and makes it more likely to spike your blood sugar. Half a cup of fresh cranberries, for example, contains just 2 grams of sugar, but half a cup of Craisins (sweetened dried cranberries) contains 58 grams! To upgrade your afternoon snack, simply choose whole fruit whenever possible. When you do choose dried fruit, be sure to seek out the kind without added sugar, and rely upon the sweet taste from the fruit itself.

11. **FRUIT JUICES:** I recall a childhood summer when I became strangely obsessed with Chex Mix and Hi-C Fruit Punch. Each time we went grocery shopping, I looked forward to restocking my supply, and enjoyed diving in as soon as we

got home. My obsession wasn't so strange after all, though, as it was likely a sugar addiction: Regularly feeding my body with pure sugar made me crave more and more sugar. The Hi-C Fruit Punch that I was hooked on lists high fructose corn syrup and sugar as its second and third ingredients after water, and contains 27 grams (nearly 7 teaspoons) of sugar per cup. Unfortunately, many juice products marketed to kids are similar in composition. To upgrade your juice intake, I recommend serving kids (and yourself!) water on almost all occasions. Transitioning kids to water by diluting juice with higher and higher portions of water can help their taste buds adjust. Creating fruit-infused waters, as we discussed in Chapter Two, can be a fun activity for the family, and can help kids appreciate the unsweetened taste of water over their usual, sugar-filled juice products.

12. **BREAD**: Adding sugar to bread provides food for the yeast to do its work, and enhances the texture. Still, many bread manufacturers go overboard, making a simple sandwich add up to a few teaspoons' worth of sugar (and that's before the barbecue sauce!). Pepperidge Farm's Whole Grain Honey Wheat bread contains 4 grams of added sugar per slice, and lists 5 versions of sweeteners in its ingredients. To upgrade your bread, I recommend choosing a bread that does not list sugar (or any of its other approved names) in the first three ingredients, and contains at least 3 grams of fiber per serving. There are many commercially-prepared wrap options coming into the marketplace that list vegetables as their primary ingredients, and don't contain any added flour or sugar (I like Raw Wraps or Wrawps). You can also try wrapping your sandwich fillings in large lettuce leaves, or thinking outside the traditional bread-filled lunch to other options like salads, soups, stews, and tasting plates.

13. **COFFEE DRINKS:** Thankfully, coffee drinks have come under fire in the media lately for being unhealthy and laden with sugar, but consumers still drool over seasonal coffee shop offerings and "can't live without" their sugar-filled go-to option each morning. The amount of sugar in many drinks at popular coffee chains is a clear illustration of why America is in such a health crisis today (and I don't say that lightly). The commercial "food" supply regularly confronts us with added sugar, chemicals, hydrogenated fats, and other unhealthy additives, and the coffee shop is no exception. The large Frozen Sugar Cookie Coffee Coolatta (made with skim milk) at Dunkin' Donuts contains 141 grams of sugar, or over 35 teaspoons. The Venti Peppermint White Chocolate Mocha at Starbucks contains 108 grams. Surely, the consumers who choose one of these options are not thinking they're making the healthiest possible decision, but they probably aren't anticipating that they are consuming over 5 days' worth of added sugar in one sweet cup. To upgrade your coffee shop choice, a simple coffee or tea is your best bet, and contains no sugar. If that's going too far, try a simple latte ... a Starbucks Grande Caffe Latte with coconut milk contains just 8 grams of sugar, and the version made with nonfat milk contains just 11 grams. Better yet, save your money and brew a nice cup of coffee or tea yourself! My office always contains a wide variety of teas, both to make the experience welcoming for clients and to stave off my own afternoon munchies in a delicious and sugar-free way!

14. **SWEET TEA:** It may seem obvious given the name, but many of my Texas-born-and-bred clients don't even realize that this Southern staple is a sugar nightmare. A large sweet tea at McDonald's contains 71 grams of added sugar, and 16 ounces of the Lipton bottled version contains 46 grams. Even

if it's not labeled as "Sweet Tea," prepared iced teas are often sweetened, so be sure to check the label before you drink. To upgrade your tea, simply choose unsweetened tea and add a squeeze of lemon juice. If the transition is too tough, start by adding stevia, then gradually reduce until you enjoy the taste of plain tea.

15. **FROZEN MEALS:** By now, it probably seems that you can't catch a break ... many of the healthy-sounding foods you may be used to choosing are loaded with sugar! Unfortunately, the TV dinners that many rely on as seemingly healthy options when there is no time to cook often are packed with the sweet stuff as well. Sugar can help preserve taste throughout the freezing process, so many manufacturers add it in generously. Even the healthier-sounding brands can have too much sugar – Weight Watchers Teriyaki Chicken & Vegetables meal contains 17 grams of sugar. When you need or want to rely on a frozen meal option, use your sugar sleuthing skills discussed earlier in the chapter to choose versions with minimal or no added sugar.

Becoming a Sugar Sleuth

While I have outlined my top 15 sources of hidden sugar here, I encourage you to become a sugar sleuth and start checking your labels for added sugar. Don't just look at the Nutrition Facts panel, where you'll see the grams of total sugar in each serving (alongside fat, protein, fiber, and more). The total sugar may include both added sugar and naturally occurring sugar, so it doesn't tell the whole story. For example, if an apple had a Nutrition Facts panel, it would tell you that it had 19 grams of sugar. The Nutrition Facts panel of a serving of Milk Duds would list the same 19 grams of sugar. However, you know from earlier in the chapter that the 19 grams of added sugar in the Milk Duds are more detrimental to your health. So how do you differentiate between these two options?

Focus your attention on the ingredient list, and look for sugar that is not naturally occurring. For example, the first ingredient on the Milk Duds is "corn syrup," followed by "sugar." Later in the ingredient list, you'll find "dextrose" and "brown sugar" as well. Anything including "sugar," "syrup," or anything ending in "-ose" is generally an added sugar ingredient.

You can gauge how much added sugar is included in a product by assessing where the sugar ingredient falls in the list of all ingredients. Ingredients must be listed in descending order of predominance by weight, so the product contains a lot of the first ingredient in the list, and much less of the last ingredient in the list. In general, if sugar (or another word for sugar) falls in the first three ingredients of a product that is not supposed to be sweet, it is something I recommend avoiding. Regularly choosing bread, cereal, sauces, or other products that include sugar in the first three ingredients increases the likelihood of taking in more added sugar than your body can effectively handle.

Salt: Equally as Deadly as Sugar?

Just as our intake of sugar has skyrocketed, so has our intake of salt, and most Americans now consume more than twice the recommended intake of sodium each day. So, is our sodium intake just as worrisome as our sugar intake, from a health perspective?

It may surprise you to hear that I don't make my clients throw away their salt shakers, and I'm not quite as concerned with sodium intake as I am with sugar intake, for most people.

Here's the main reason: if we're eating mostly unpackaged, unrefined foods, we will automatically limit our sodium intake to an acceptable level. It's important to note that if you aim to limit your sodium intake, the place to start is with packaged foods. In fact, even if you use the salt shaker regularly, only 6 percent of your intake of sodium is likely to be from the salt you add to your food at the table! About 5 percent is added during cooking, and a whopping 77 percent is from restaurant or processed food.[52] (The remaining percentage comes from the sodium that is naturally occurring in foods.) So, even if you add a few sprinkles of salt on the broccoli you cook at home, you're still coming in far under the sodium you'd take in if you had a similar side dish at a restaurant.

Why should you care about your sodium intake, anyway? Sodium is critical for your survival and health, especially if you exercise regularly. Sodium and potassium work together to manage your blood pressure, generate nerve and muscle impulses, and help with nutrient absorption. So, a diet containing some sodium is a very good thing.

For most people, any excess sodium taken in is simply excreted by the body, either in sweat output, or through the urine. However, in some people (who are called "salt sensitive"), excess sodium intake is correlated with increased blood pressure, which is a risk factor for both stroke and heart disease. There are many factors associated with hypertension, including smoking and being overweight, so we cannot say that sodium intake alone is responsible for hypertension. However, if you have hypertension (another word for high blood pressure), it's not a bad idea to monitor your sodium intake, and see if your condition improves after a few months on a low-sodium diet.

As you have learned to check labels for added sugar, you can now check out the sodium content as well. If a packaged meal has more than 30 percent of your RDA for sodium, or a snack has more than 15 percent of your RDA for sodium, you may be better off choosing a different option. If you are otherwise healthy, and you choose a diet that is limited in processed and refined foods, though, a little bit of salt from the shaker is a tasty – and healthy – way to amplify the flavor in your food.

~ Recipe: Zucchini Apple Breakfast Muffins ~

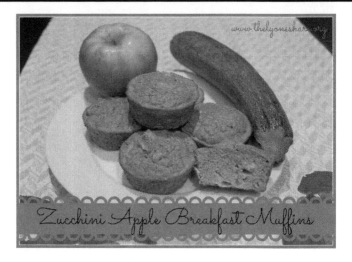

Most of us don't get vegetables with breakfast, but with these healthy muffins, you'll sneak in multiple fruits and vegetables!

Makes 9 muffins. Each muffin will contain 72 calories, 1g fat, 12g carbs, and 5g protein (depending on the protein powder used). What's best ... only 5 grams of sugar each!

INGREDIENTS

½ – ⅔ cup of grated zucchini (about 140g)

½ large apple (any kind will work, I prefer Gala for this recipe; the half-apple should be about 150g)

½ cup of egg whites (or 3 large egg whites, or 2 large whole eggs)

¼ cup of canned pumpkin (not pumpkin pie filling)

2 Tbsp. of unsweetened applesauce

½ cup of quinoa flour (quinoa flour is a medium-bodied, gluten-free, slightly-higher-in-protein flour that I often use for baking, but feel free to substitute other types of flour here if you prefer)

1 scoop (about 32g) of vanilla flavored protein powder

1.5 tsp. cinnamon

1 tsp. vanilla extract

2 tsp. pumpkin pie spice

1 tsp. baking powder

¼ tsp. salt

2 Tbsp. xylitol (a naturally-occurring sweetener that's lower in calories than sugar, although you could use sugar or another sweetener if you prefer). The xylitol, protein powder, apple, and applesauce should provide enough sweetness for the muffins, but if your protein powder is unsweetened, you may choose to increase the xylitol or add a few teaspoons of stevia to compensate.

INSTRUCTIONS

Preheat oven to 350 degrees.

Grate your zucchini into a large bowl. Blot or pat dry, but don't squeeze out the extra liquid.

Add in egg whites, pumpkin, applesauce, and vanilla, and stir gently to combine.

In a separate bowl, mix dry ingredients (protein powder, flour, spice, salt, baking powder, and sweetener).

Pour dry ingredients into wet ingredients, and stir to form a batter.

Chop apples into small pieces, and sprinkle a little bit of extra flour on top, until apples are just coated (this helps the apples stay distributed throughout the muffins, rather than sinking to the bottom).

Fold apples into batter and gently stir to combine.

Distribute batter among 9 muffin cups, sprayed with oil or cooking spray.

Bake for 20 minutes at 350 degrees, and enjoy!

Chapter Five

You've Got to Move It

Finding Motivation and Joy in Exercise

If you don't exercise regularly right now, you probably cringe when people say things like, "I just LOVE waking up at 5 a.m. to work out." The "high" of exercise is something you truly don't understand until you get into the habit of doing it regularly, and (let's be honest), it just doesn't feel quite as good the first few times you do it. If you haven't gone for a run in a few years, things are going to jiggle that didn't used to jiggle, you'll run out of breath much more quickly than you expect, and your form is going to feel awkward. If you haven't been to the gym in many months, you're not going to be able to lift the same amount of weight that you're used to, and you may not even remember your regular routine. If you haven't set your alarm for the wee hours of the morning in a while, chances are you're going to question your sanity when it starts ringing, and play some mental jiujitsu to rationalize that it's probably the better decision to just stay in bed.

But if you do convince yourself to put one foot in front of the other, continue lifting the lighter weights until you can build up your strength to get back to the heavy weights, and just get out of bed and get moving, you'll find that, over time, the habit becomes engrained as part of your daily routine that you actually look forward to, not one you dread every single time.

There is scientific rationale for this – endorphins, the chemicals that make you feel good, are actually released with many types of exercise. You may have heard of the "runner's high," and there is truth behind the catchy name. Many people do, in fact, feel jubilant when they exercise for long enough to get that rush of pleasure chemicals in the brain.

Aside from the science, I'll tell you from personal experience that the joy of a regular exercise routine goes beyond the actual time in which you are moving. Going to workout classes and running in races, feeling fit and in shape, and knowing that I dedicate time nearly every day to take care of my body and my health all add up to make exercise a critically important part of my life. If I go for several days in a row without a workout, my close friends and family probably know that something is "off," because I'm simply not as happy and relaxed when I haven't been exercising.

I love the feeling that I *can* physically run up a flight of stairs, sprint after a bus, or even enter a half marathon because I am already fit and active. I love that exercising is a time to truly disconnect – I'm not knee-deep in my email inbox, I'm not staring at my to-do list, and I'm not feeling guilty that I'm not in the office. I love that, if there is something to think about, it somehow gets resolved much more easily if I'm on a run or in a yoga class. Most of all, though, I love that I can challenge myself every single day and know that I'm taking steps to make myself just a bit better than I was the day before.

That's a peek into my personal motivation to exercise, but you need to find what motivates *you* uniquely. To get you started, here are eleven reasons why exercise can benefit your overall health and well-being.

Eleven Reasons a Regular Exercise Routine Will Improve Your Health

- IT WILL HELP YOU LIVE A LONGER, HEALTHIER LIFE: It's generally hard for us to focus on doing something now when the benefits are intangible and not instantaneous. If you don't exercise today, it doesn't mean that you're going to have a heart attack tomorrow, or the next day, or even the next year. Still, thinking about how your healthy lifestyle will improve your quantity *and quality* of life can be motivating and exciting.

  Just think about Faujah Singh, who started running marathons in his late-80s. When he was 99, his medical tests showed that he "was a man of 40 years of age." He retired from marathons at 101 years old, but continues to run and walk daily because it makes him happy and keeps him healthy.[53] Now *that* is the kind of aging we can aspire to!

  In a 2004 study, researchers showed a more than 50 percent reduction in mortality from any cause associated with being fit and active.[54] A similar study showed that middle-aged women who did not exercise (or who performed less than one hour of exercise per week) had a 52 percent increase in risk of dying from any cause. The researchers estimated that reducing excess weight and reversing physical inactivity could prevent 31 percent of all premature deaths.[55] To put it simply: You can cut your risk of dying in half, simply by staying physically fit. I'll gladly trade a small portion of every day to increase my chances of living a longer, happier, and healthier life, and I think you're selling yourself short if you don't choose the same.

- **IT HAS INCREDIBLE BENEFITS FOR YOUR HEART.** It is frequently discussed in health news, so you probably have heard that exercise is good for your heart. Exercise has long been touted as the best method of preventing heart disease, and for good reason. Physical activity can increase your HDL ("good" cholesterol), lower your triglycerides, and help prevent heart disease, high blood pressure, and stroke. The middle-aged, inactive women in the previously mentioned study had *double* the risk of dying from cardiovascular issues compared with the physically active group.[56] Even those who already have heart disease showed dramatic decreases in risk of dying when they started (and committed to) an exercise program![57]

There's no better way to keep your heart healthy than to get it pumping as regularly as possible. Just like your biceps grow stronger when you lift weights regularly, your heart gets stronger each time it has to work hard. To get the benefits, you don't have to feel like your heart is going to burst out of your chest; you just have to elevate your heart rate a bit – enough that you feel slightly short of breath (about the pace of a brisk walk). Of course, higher intensity exercise has fantastic cardiac benefits as well. So if you are physically able, adding in some heart-pumping cardio is a great idea.

- **IT CAN HELP PREVENT DIABETES.** An amazing study showed that every 500 calories burned during exercise each week reduced the risk of Type 2 diabetes by six percent in participants (up to 3,500 calories a week).[58] This is an incredible finding, and shows in no uncertain terms that exercising does reduce risk for Type 2 diabetes, even in those already at high-risk for diabetes. And 500 calories a week is about the equivalent of walking 4-5 miles a week, for an average person. If that seems like too much, even 40 minutes a week of moderate-level physical activity has been proven to be effective in preventing Type 2 diabetes.

For those at high risk for Type 2 diabetes (including those who are overweight or have a family history of Type 2 diabetes), losing weight and starting an exercise program can result in a reduction of 40-60 percent in the incidence of diabetes in just 3-4 years.[59] Upping that to 150 minutes a week of physical activity was even more effective than Metformin, a prescription medication that is commonly prescribed to help prevent and manage Type 2 diabetes.[60]

Let me just re-emphasize: *Exercise is more effective than prescription medication in preventing and managing Type 2 diabetes!*

For those who already have Type 2 diabetes, exercise continues to be helpful in extending both quality and quantity of life. Walking at least two hours a week was associated with a 39-54 percent reduction in death from any cause in those who have Type 2 diabetes. Just four, 30-minute strolls around the neighborhood each week (or 17 minutes per day) could keep you alive longer!

• **PREVENTING OTHER ILLNESSES.** In addition to heart disease and diabetes, exercise has been proven effective in preventing a wide number of other illnesses. The same middle-aged, inactive women we've mentioned twice also had a 29 percent increase in cancer-related mortality compared with the women who exercised regularly.[61] Colon cancer and breast cancer are particularly influenced by physical activity, and the reduction in cancer recurrence and risk of death for women with either of those cancers can be up to 40 percent with physical activity.[62] While we haven't been able to pinpoint exactly what causes many types of cancer, a significant difference in risk forms a compelling enough reason for me to keep pounding the pavement!

Bone loss, osteoporosis, and fractures are dramatically reduced with a regular exercise program, and exercise can reduce bone loss. The benefits of exercise extend to prevention and treatment of many other conditions as well, including arthritis, asthma, back pain, fatty liver and other liver disease, and more. In short, being active and fit in general is associated with a more than 50 percent reduction in the risk of death from all causes.[63] That's a significant reason to get moving!

- **IT INCREASES YOUR ENERGY AND ENHANCES YOUR MOOD.** If you're feeling lethargic and tired, it can be easy to rationalize sleeping in, rather than setting your alarm early to get to the gym. However, getting your heart pumping actually gives you more energy throughout the day! By getting freshly oxygenated blood flowing throughout your body, we immediately feel refreshed and more awake after exercise. Unless you are severely sleep-deprived, 10 minutes of exercise will energize you more than an additional 10 minutes of sleep.

It is also frequently noted that exercise provides an endorphin rush, which gives you the "feel good" sensation that lasts for several hours after the actual exercise session. Plus, the sense of pride and accomplishment experienced after completing an exercise session casts a positive light on the rest of the day. I always remind myself that I can get a head start on a chaotic day by ensuring that I get in my exercise first thing in the morning. That way, no matter what the day throws at me, I already will have accomplished something important to me and to my health.

- **IT ENHANCES SELF-CONFIDENCE.** I can tell you from personal experience (and from research)[64] that when people are in a regular exercise routine, their self-confidence and self-image are dramatically improved. For me and for the many clients I have seen experience this positive side effect of exercise, there is something about committing to a regular exercise routine that not only produces a sense of accomplishment, but also leads to appreciation of the body's abilities, and even improvements in the way we criticize (or appreciate) the way we look.

- **IT CAN LOWER STRESS, ANXIETY, AND DEPRESSION.** Quite simply, when you feel better about yourself, have more energy, and are physically healthier, your mental health will improve as well. Numerous studies have shown the benefits of exercise on stress, anxiety, and depression, and exercise is now a widely recognized treatment for depression. Some research even shows that, for some patients, exercise is more reliable and effective than traditional medications for depression.[65] Of course, if you are dealing with clinical depression, I highly recommend that you seek appropriate treatment. But I think an exercise program as part of that treatment can be a great benefit. And if you find yourself stressed and anxious more than you'd like, consider giving exercise a try. What better reason to exercise than living a happier life?

- **IT BOOSTS MEMORY FUNCTION.** Many studies show that exercise increases memory in both the short-term and the long-term. One such study, done in 2013, showed significant improvement on memory tests after just six months of aerobic training or resistance training (although the aerobic training group showed slightly more positive results).[66] We could all use some improved memory!

- **IT INCREASES PRODUCTIVITY.** I can detect a definite difference in my stress level and productivity at work between days when I've exercised in the morning and days that I haven't. Sometimes, when I find myself procrastinating on a project or having writer's block, I force myself to do 20 jumping jacks, go for a quick walk around the block, or even do a few handstands to get the blood flowing to my head. Maybe it's the break in routine just as much as the actual activity, but I know this works wonders for me, and I'm confident the impact is replicable.

  Studies show that when employers force their employees to take a break and exercise, productivity stays the same or increases (despite fewer hours worked).[67] Encouraging employees to exercise (via flexible hours, gym facilities in the building, discounts on gyms included in workers' benefits, walking meetings, etc.) benefits the company bottom line, and I'm confident that more and more employers will begin moving this way in the near future.

- **IT ENHANCES YOUR SLEEP QUALITY.** There's absolutely nothing like a great night of sleep, and exercising during the day is one way to help yourself achieve it. A 2011 study showed that people who exercised 150 minutes a week (just 22 minutes per day!) had a 65 percent improvement in sleep, and felt significantly less tired during the day.[68] Exercising at a regular time in the morning can help your body regulate its natural circadian rhythms, making you tired and ready for bed in the evening. Although research is mixed, I encourage you to not exercise 1-2 hours before bed, as the impact may be the opposite, given exercise's potential to energize you right away.

- **It helps manage or maintain body weight.** This may be the most commonly touted reason to exercise, but I encourage you to not think of it as the *only* reason to exercise. In fact, people who say their motivation to exercise is to feel good actually have better success than people whose only motivation is to lose weight. When the going gets tough, it's harder for us to be motivated by the idea of being at an ideal weight in the future than it is for us to be motivated by how we will feel in just 30 minutes, after our exercise session.

That said, exercise is, of course, a powerful way to help achieve a comfortable weight. It's a great way to burn calories, build muscle, and reduce fat. Just walking one mile a day (about 15-20 minutes) will help the average person burn 100 additional calories a day, or 35,600 calories per year, which equates to more than 10 pounds lost (all other factors held equal).

Even if you're not trying to lose weight, exercise is helpful in controlling your weight and keeping your body toned. You may have heard that muscle weighs more than fat, since muscle tissue is denser and more compact. So, even when people stay the same weight on the scale as they begin an exercise program, they may shrink in waist size as their muscle composition increases and the amount of body fat decreases. For this reason (and because it can get obsessive and controlling), I often encourage clients to have goals aside from just the reading on the scale. If your favorite jeans fit more comfortably after a month of eating healthily and exercising, you're moving in the right direction, regardless of what the scale reads.

How Much Is Enough

Now that you know that exercise is one of the best things you can do for your health, how much is enough? Many of the studies referenced in this chapter use 3.5 hours per week of moderate-intensity activity as a baseline. This means that your heart rate needs to be elevated for approximately 30 minutes a day. This doesn't mean that you need to be *running* 30 minutes a day, or work yourself to physical exhaustion (although bursts of higher intensity are definitely helpful for weight loss!). It just means you need to get moving. Taking a few laps around your office building, going up and down the stairs multiple times each day, or walking as you do a quick errand can all count toward your 30 minutes. If you start paying attention to adding in a little bit of movement here and there, the minutes will add up quickly.

If 30 minutes a day seems like a huge stretch for you, I encourage you to start small. Breaking big goals down into small chunks is one of the most effective ways I've found of helping people take action. You may not have time or energy to start with 30 minutes right off the bat, but could you give me *one* minute? I have no doubt that even the busiest person can find a single minute to exercise. Simply commit to doing one minute of exercise tomorrow (try jumping jacks or lunges), then add on one minute every single day. In just a month, you'll be exercising 30 minutes a day, without ever feeling overwhelmed or taking a big leap.

You can't train for a marathon in a day; you can't get to your ideal body or fitness level in a day; and you can't become an exercise "regular" in a day. So have patience with yourself! If you're at the beginning of your exercise journey; start slowly and build until you get to approximately 30 minutes every day.

If, on the other hand, you're already exercising regularly, it may be time for you to bump it up a notch. Maybe you walk for 30 minutes each day, but you could try running for a few minutes, or extend your walk to 45 minutes on a weekend day. Maybe you fit in two yoga classes each week, but could squeeze in an extra one if you recorded your favorite TV show and watched it on the weekend instead. Maybe you're used to driving to work, but you could start walking or biking. Whatever your situation, take this as motivation to honestly assess whether you would benefit from moving just a bit more often.

The truly "perfect" amount of exercise will vary for each person, but as a general rule, I recommend at least 3 exercise sessions a week for someone who is otherwise fairly sedentary (working a desk job, for example). If you'd rather not get in official exercise sessions, but will be active during the day, I recommend going beyond the 30 minutes used in studies and tallying at least 45 minutes of movement per day (if you're a parent of a small child, for example, you're likely moving all throughout the day. In this case, if you rack up at least 45 minutes of active time, such as when you are walking with your child in a stroller or playing on the playground with your child, you will meet the requirement). For most Americans, more exercise is better, so unless you are already exerting yourself regularly, I encourage you to find ways to increase your activity level.

How to Find What You Love

Now that you're (hopefully) convinced to get moving, do you have to sign up for a gym membership and slog away on the elliptical every single day? No! The days of the traditional gym facility are waning with the advent of boutique fitness studios, outdoor exercise classes, at-home workout options, and non-traditional forms of exercise. In fact, I haven't had a traditional gym membership for years, and I'm just as fit as ever!

One key to keeping yourself motivated to exercise is finding something you enjoy. To do this, think about what you liked to do as a child. Were you always dancing around the house, participating in school musicals, or listening to music? Maybe a Zumba class would be a good fit for you! Were you constantly running around your back yard, faster than your parents could chase after you? Maybe walking or running would still make you happy! Did you thrive on team sports like soccer or basketball? Adult sports leagues are more popular now than ever! Did you constantly wrestle with your siblings, or find ways to get your aggression out? A kickboxing class or karate lesson may give you the same release today! Were you a water baby? Adult swim classes – or even triathlons – are a fantastic way to get in your movement! Even if you say, "I really hated everything physical; I just wanted to get through recess to get back to math class," you can take a lesson from your childhood. Maybe you didn't like recess because you felt judged or because you prefer recharging alone. How about something like cycling, where you are alone with the road and your thoughts for hours on end?

If you don't like the first few things you try, don't get discouraged. Keep going, and you will eventually find something that you love. These days, monthly fitness subscriptions like ClassPass (or StudioHop in Texas) allow members to try a variety of classes from boutique studios (like yoga, spinning, dance, kickboxing, and general fitness studios) by paying one monthly membership fee. This can be a great way to find what you enjoy without breaking the bank.

There are many fitness studios that offer a variety of classes all in one studio. If you happen to be in Dallas, Dallas Grit Fitness offers a full variety of classes, all of which are music-driven, energizing, and fun, and has a welcoming community feel.

Once you find what you love (for now), continue checking in with yourself regularly. You may get in the yoga groove for a few months, then suddenly realize you're craving more intensity. You may be all about spinning classes, until you realize that you're no longer feeling excited to saddle up each morning and a change would do you good. Changing your preferences is normal, and as long as you find your new exercise love before you fall out of the routine of exercise altogether, you're no worse for the wear.

The goal should be to feel more energized, physically and mentally, after each exercise session, and to look forward to the next time you can lace up your sneakers. If you haven't yet found something that gives you that feeling, keep looking. With experimentation and persistence, you *will* find what you love.

Making Exercise a Habit

Once you achieve the mentality that exercise is a critical part of your day, find something you love doing, and feel motivated to incorporate it regularly, you're much more likely to create a *habit* of regular exercise. If you treat it as a reward you're giving yourself, rather than a punishment you're inflicting upon yourself, it can become something you look forward to. You may even find yourself feeling "off" if you skip exercise for a few days in a row, feeling anxious for your next exercise session, or wishing you were exercising instead of doing whatever you happen to be doing at the time. When any of these things happen, congratulations! You have gotten into the habit of exercising regularly.

One of my absolute favorite things is to observe friends and family who are beginning (or re-starting) their exercise journey. For the first several days, it's an obvious internal battle, and they have to "force themselves" to exercise. Slowly but surely, though, they turn the corner and get hooked on the endorphin rush, self-confidence, and energy burst that exercise provides ... and soon, exercise is a habit for them, as well!

You've probably heard the concept that it takes 21 days to form a new habit (although some studies show that it varies widely between 18 and 254 days). So, if exercise is not a regular part of your life, don't get discouraged if it still feels like a struggle a few days or weeks into your journey. It can take time, and that's OK. Here are a few quick and easy tips to help you turn exercise into habit:

- **DO SOME PLANNING.** If you map out when you'll spend time exercising during every day of the upcoming week, you'll be much more likely to stick to it. Will you hit spin class after work on Tuesday? Go for a run on Thursday morning? Identify what suits your schedule, and literally make a note in your calendar. You are much more likely to honor the commitment if it is scheduled just like any other appointment, and if you take it just as seriously. Of course, things come up, and that's OK - if your body is telling you that you need a rest day, or if a serious conflict gets in the way, you can reschedule your exercise. Just be honest about what a serious conflict is!

- **SET OUT YOUR CLOTHES THE NIGHT BEFORE.** It seems like a simple step, but having everything ready to go before you need to hit the road can be very helpful. Some people like to sleep in their workout clothes; others like to put their shoes by the bathroom door so they'll stumble over them. Whatever option works for you is great; just be sure to make it easy to get out the door without making excuses or delaying.

- **USE SOCIAL MEDIA TO MOTIVATE YOU!** Apps like *MapMyRun*, *MyFitnessPal*, *Sparkpeople*, *DailyMile* can help you track your progress and share it with others. If you have a step tracker like a FitBit, you can be "friends" with others and compare progress to keep your motivation high. Although I am not prone to posting every workout on Facebook, I often post a race time to Instagram, and feel proud when I get positive feedback. Of course, when I see friends' status updates sharing their own progress, I love encouraging them with a simple "like" of their status! Won't you feel great about yourself if your whole social network is cheering you on?

- **FIND A FRIEND AND EXERCISE WITH HIM OR HER!** Tell each other you'll meet for a morning class at the gym, or walk to a meeting place between your houses. If you're in a new location, search for a local running club or activity group. Having others around you with the same goal can be very motivating!

If you don't have an in-person friend, or want additional accountability, join the Start Here Community – the most supportive and encouraging accountability community on Facebook! Simply go to **www.StartHereCommunity.com** and request to join.

- **CHEER YOURSELF ON.** Give yourself a small reward, or at least mentally recognize the progress you're making. Look for small, midpoint goals, and celebrate them. It can be so easy to beat ourselves up, rather than focus on the positive. Instead, be proud of the days that you get in some activity!

- **THINK ABOUT HOW YOU'LL FEEL AFTERWARDS.** I never regret a workout after the fact, and I love the burst of energy it provides. So, if I'm struggling to get going, I envision where I'll be a few hours into the future and how great I'll feel after having worked out.

- **SET A "TRIGGER" TO CHECK IN WITH YOURSELF.** Every time you brush your teeth, or go to the coffee maker, or whatever else you choose ... think about how you'll fit in exercise the following day. Keeping it top-of-mind will help you on your way!

Striking the Right Balance

As a runner, I hear a *lot* of people say that focusing on anything else other than running is a waste of time. Both my husband and my father-in-law are fantastic runners, and they do very little aside from just running. In fact, even in my running coaching training (held by Road Runner's Club of America, a nationally recognized running coach training), I was told that cross training (any activity other than running) was detrimental, and that a runner should just focus on running.

I run the risk of ruffling many feathers here, but I feel strongly about this: For most people, *it's just not true.* Sure, there are some people whose bodies are cut out to run (or to lift weights, or to do some other singular activity), and for these people, spending time on any other activity is just taking time away from the goal. Even some Olympic athletes choose to do just one type of training, and do it a lot without getting injured frequently. If you are in this camp, consider yourself lucky.

But the vast majority of people need balance in their training, and run the risk of mental and physical burnout if they do not vary their routines regularly. When you focus on one activity, the muscles used during that activity get stronger. Let's say you love spinning classes; your quadriceps muscles are getting a great workout. This is a good thing, until you consider potential muscle imbalances. Your hamstrings (the back side of your upper leg) are not getting as much of a workout as your quadriceps during a spinning class, and the resulting imbalance can lead to posture and gait changes.

When I focused primarily on running for a few years, I was constantly battling some nagging pain or minor injury, until I began incorporating strength training, yoga, boot camp, and even walking. My upper body was decidedly weak (have you ever noticed how many Olympic marathon runners have needle-like, weak arms?), and while I could run, I certainly was not what I would call "fit." Now, through a variety of types of exercise, particularly my bootcamp classes at Jay Johnson's Bootcamp in Dallas (which require a variety of skills and incorporate cardiovascular, strength, plyometric, balance, and endurance drills), I feel more fit when I'm trading some of the running for cross-training, and better yet, I perform better in running, too!

It's not just me – even the most successful athletes have found that incorporating cross training makes them stronger overall, and helps prevent injuries. Michael Phelps, the world record holder and winner of 22 individual Olympic medals, reportedly includes weight lifting, sled pulling, boxing, running, and stretching in his regular exercise routine. Olympic middle-distance runner Nick Symmonds is a vocal advocate of varying workouts, and he incorporates weight training, swimming, and cycling into his training program. LeBron James, one of the most dominant NBA players in history, includes yoga, Pilates, boxing, cycling, sprinting, weightlifting, and stretching in his conditioning plan.

Chances are, though, that if you're reading this book, you're not training to be an Olympic athlete. Neither am I! You're still not off the hook, though. Although you may not have to be quite as rigid in developing a balanced plan, it's still important to include variety in your exercise routine. Maybe that means going to one Body Pump class each week, attending one yoga class, and getting in two walks or runs. Maybe that means a bit of stretching on days that you're not riding your bike. Whatever it means for you, I encourage you to focus on conditioning multiple muscle groups, including both cardio and strength training, and balancing intensity with flexibility.

The All-or-Nothing Mentality

It's very common for my clients to want to get back on track with exercising. When I ask them what they want to achieve in the upcoming week, they'll say casually, "oh, I plan to hit the gym for an hour every day after work, then I'll just do a really long walk on Saturday." That may be a great plan for someone who has been exercising consistently for years, but for someone who is just starting (or restarting) a program, that's a sure recipe for failure!

While it's tempting to fall into the all-or-nothing mentality and think that you're either "on" an exercise program or "off" it, that thinking is counterproductive and unrealistic. If you're just starting, ease into it. You might want to start with 5 minutes, two times the first week, and increase gradually. If that seems like too little to be beneficial, consider this: *The Journal of the American College of Cardiology* found that just 5 minutes of leisure running a day is enough to lower your risk of death from cardiovascular disease by 45 percent![69]

If you find yourself thinking "I skipped yesterday's workout, so I'm already off the plan. I'll just start over next week," then remind yourself how illogical that is. Just because you skipped yesterday's workout does not mean that tomorrow's workout will be less beneficial. In fact, it may be even more important to get in that workout tomorrow! So, consider every opportunity a new chance to restart. There's simply no room for black-and-white, all-or-nothing thinking when it comes to your health

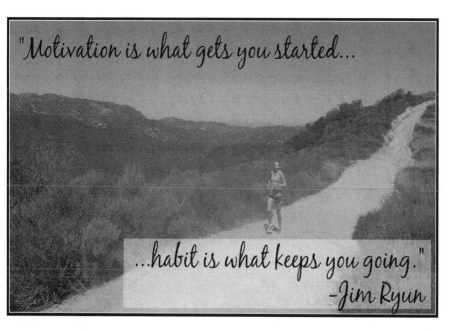

"Motivation is what gets you started...

...habit is what keeps you going."
-Jim Ryun

Greasing the Groove

I first heard of the concept of "Greasing the Groove" from Ben Greenfield, a fitness and lifestyle performance coach and the brains (and brawn!) behind the Ben Greenfield Fitness podcast. It seemed like a fantastic way to incorporate exercise into a daily routine without giving up a large chunk of time, and it's worked great for me and for several of my clients since then. Basically, Ben's adapted concept is that you form a habit of performing a small number of repetitions of a given exercise multiple times throughout the day.

As far as I can tell, the initial concept was created by Pavel Tsatsouline in his book, *The Naked Warrior*. He created "greasing the groove" because he believed that "Specificity + Frequent Practice = Success" ... that being able to achieve a strength goal is not only based on building overall muscle bulk, but also based on practicing that specific activity frequently. For a while, it was mostly used by bodybuilders ... an easy way to achieve a goal of bench-pressing 300 pounds, say, was to bench-press 150 pounds several times a day. (And no, I cannot and will never have a desire to bench press 300 pounds, so this does not apply to only body-builders!)

Here's a quote from Ben that explains the benefits well:

> *This concept works because by performing a movement frequently, your neuromuscular system becomes more proficient at allowing your body, your nerves and your muscles to work in sync to perform that movement more efficiently, and over time the movement becomes more natural and more economical for your body to perform. When that happens, you're able to maintain better form and do more repetitions.*[70]

Think about how this may apply to your situation ... if you create a habit of doing a tiny bit of exercise that would otherwise seem inconsequential, you'll end up fitting in a whole lot more exercise during a regular day than you otherwise would have, without ever spending more than 60 seconds on an activity or feeling like you're really working out. Doesn't that sound like a win-win situation?

One example that I have borrowed from Ben is doing 20 squats every time I use the restroom. (And if you're following the tips from Chapter Two on hydration, you'll be using this one frequently!) While 20 squats at a time may not be a challenge in itself, I'm certain that adding 200 squats to every day will make anyone's legs stronger and leaner! When I'm in the habit of doing this, I can tell that it makes a big difference in my strength.

Here are several other exercises you could include in your "Greasing the Groove" routine:

GREASING THE GROOVE

EVERY TIME I ...	I WILL DO ...
- Use the restroom	- 20 squats
- Pick up the phone	- Stand up or walk
-Open the fridge	-25 jumping jacks
-Brush my teeth	-30 calf raises
-Check Facebook	- 15 push-ups
-Turn on the TV	-1 minute plank

WWW.THELYONSSHARE.ORG

1. Standing or walking each time you pick up the phone

2. Doing 25 jumping jacks each time you open the refrigerator

3. Doing 30 calf raises each time you brush your teeth

4. Doing 15 pushups each time you check Facebook

5. Doing 1 burpee each time you walk in the door of your office

6. Holding a plank for 1 minute each time you turn on the TV

7. Running up and down the stairs before you sit down to dinner

Doesn't that look easy? I encourage you to start with just one or two, so that you actually remember them and they don't put an undue burden on your day. Be sure to adjust the number of reps to something that is not too challenging for you to do at once, but adds up when you do it throughout the day. Have fun, and enjoy getting stronger and leaner without much effort!

Standing Up for Your Health

In today's society, it's completely normal to be stuck in a chair all day. We might check our social media and email first thing in the morning, drive to work (seated, of course), spend another 8 or more hours behind a desk, and get home and relax on the couch all evening. Before I started The Lyons' Share Wellness, I tallied my computer hours, and at one point I was spending an average of 15 hours a day staring at a computer! Aside from the fact that too much screen time is generally not recommended for our brain health, just the act of sitting for a long period of time is more detrimental to our overall health than most of us realize.

Sitting for extended periods of time makes you more prone to the following 10 conditions:

HEART DAMAGE: People with the most sedentary time recorded are more than twice as likely to have cardiovascular disease than those with the least sedentary time recorded![71]

MUSCLES BURNING LESS FAT: Standing can burn up to 310 extra calories per day.[72]

OVERPRODUCTIVE PANCREAS, which could eventually lead to diabetes and several other diseases.

HIGHER RISK OF COLON, BREAST, AND ENDOMETRIAL CANCER, potentially due to increased insulin, or the lack of exercise-induced antioxidant boosts.

QUICKER MUSCLE DEGENERATION, including weaker abs, sway-back, tight hips and hip flexors, and weaker gluteus muscles.

BAD CIRCULATION IN THE LEGS, leading to varicose veins and pain.

WEAKER BONES, likely because of less exposure to the weight-bearing impact that strengthens bones.

SLOWER BRAIN FUNCTION, potentially due to the lack of stimulation that occurs when "zoning out" in front of the TV or computer.

STRAINED NECK, SORE SHOULDERS, AND BACK PAIN, due to our terrible posture when seated at a desk in front of a computer. The next time you sit at your computer, notice if your chin juts out, putting undue strain on your neck. Try to keep your computer screen at eye level, and keep your arms bent at 90 degrees. Sit up with your back supported, and don't slouch forward!

DEATH. It sounds dramatic, but the correlation between sitting and early death has been proven repeatedly. One study showed that those adults who sat for six or more hours a day had an increased risk of death during the 14-year follow-up period, all other things held equal. Unexplainably, the risk was 34 percent higher for women, and only 17 percent higher for men.[73] (I guess some things in life just aren't fair!)

Those who watched the most TV in one study had a 61 percent greater risk of dying during the study than those who watched less than one hour a day, even after controlling for age, sex, smoking status, education, diet, race, *and* physical activity![74]

Unfortunately for those of us who think we get a "free pass" to sit all day after a dedicated exercise session, the detriment of sitting for extended periods of time impacts even those who exercise regularly. Despite short bouts of actual exercise, we still succumb to the metabolic changes that inactivity and sitting can bring.

If you work in a traditional office, you're probably thinking that you're required to be sitting for much of the day, so there's nothing you can do about this particular health risk. Fortunately, more and more offices are becoming open to alternative workstations, such as standing desks, varied-height desks, and even treadmill desks! At my home office, I have an inexpensive, foldable desktop stand (available at bit.ly/AmazonStandingDesk) that raises my computer to standing height, and I try to alternate between sitting and standing there. At my office, I purchased a desk with two levels – one for sitting across from clients during health coaching, and the other to stand while on the phone or using Skype with clients, or while working on my computer. I make it a policy to stand as much as possible, and never take phone calls while seated (of course, I'm standing as I write this, as well).

If you are able to stand while on the phone, or get a standing desk to facilitate standing, I encourage you to alternate throughout the day. Try standing for 10 minutes out of every hour, or standing for half an hour in the morning and half an hour in the afternoon. Build up gradually – you may be surprised that your feet and legs can get sore simply from standing more often! Also, it is important to shift your weight or pace around a bit while standing; otherwise, you risk the same blood pooling as you would with sitting.

If standing while working is impossible, you're not off the hook. I highly recommend that you make a point to stand up every hour, even if you just have 30 seconds to take a break. For the first few days, set an alarm on your computer or phone to remind you to stand up – you'll be amazed at how long you're used to sitting without the reminder!

If you're drinking enough water, you may also require regular restroom breaks, which is a great way to force yourself to get up. If you are thinking that it's just impossible to take such regular breaks, I'll remind you that this is critical for your health, and that you have time for what you prioritize. I can think of very few job situations that would not permit even 15 seconds of standing at your desk each hour. So, commit to making it happen, and just do it!

~ Recipe: Quick at-home workouts ~

For a fun, 15-minute workout that lets you tally up 500 reps, try my **500 Reps Workout.**

For full descriptions, visit http://www.thelyonsshare. org/2013/07/17/500-rep-circuit-workout/ or Google "Lyons Share 500 Reps Workout" and click on the first result.

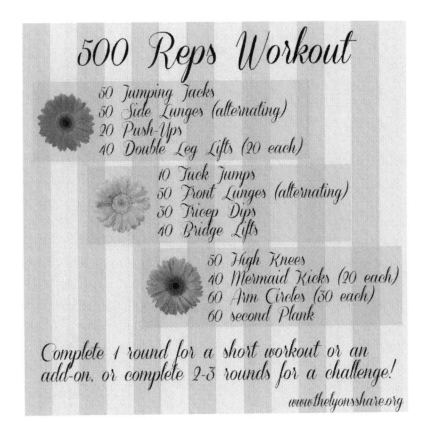

500 Reps Workout

50 Jumping Jacks
50 Side Lunges (alternating)
20 Push-Ups
40 Double Leg Lifts (20 each)

10 Tuck Jumps
50 Front Lunges (alternating)
30 Tricep Dips
40 Bridge Lifts

50 High Knees
40 Mermaid Kicks (20 each)
60 Arm Circles (30 each)
60 second Plank

Complete 1 round for a short workout or an add-on, or complete 2-3 rounds for a challenge!

www.thelyonsshare.org

For an intense, 8-minute (or 24-minutes if you repeat it three times)Tabata-style workout, try my **8-minute Tabata Workout.**

For full descriptions and a video, visit:

www.thelyonsshare.org/ 2014/05/28/8-minute-or-24- minute-full-body-tabata-work- out/ or Google "Lyons Share 8-minute Tabata" and click on the first result.

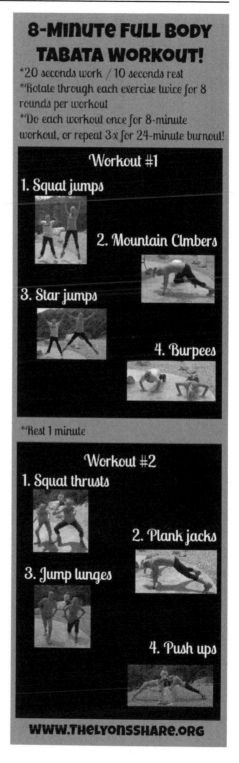

8-MINUTE FULL BODY TABATA WORKOUT!

*20 seconds work / 10 seconds rest
**Rotate through each exercise twice for 8 rounds per workout
*Do each workout once for 8-minute workout, or repeat 3x for 24-minute burnout!

Workout #1

1. Squat jumps

2. Mountain Climbers

3. Star jumps

4. Burpees

**Rest 1 minute

Workout #2
1. Squat thrusts

2. Plank jacks

3. Jump lunges

4. Push ups

WWW.THELYONSSHARE.ORG

For a fun, family-friendly workout that can be done in 15 minutes, try my **Fit-It-In Turkey Day Workout.**

For full descriptions, visit:

www.thelyonsshare.org/2013/11/27/fit-it-in-turkey-day-work-out-runners-problem-areas-thanksgiving-laughs-and-thank-you/ or Google "Lyons Share Turkey Day Workout" and click on the first result.

Asterisks in the graphic below indicate that a video demonstration is available on the website.

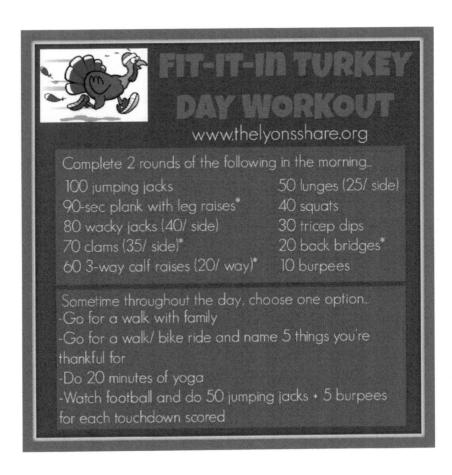

For an intense, 5-minute (plus warm-up), abdominal-focused workout, try this **Flat Abs in 5 Minutes** workout.

To find a full description, Google "Lyons Share Flat Abs 5 Minutes" and click on the first result or go to:

www.thelyonsshare.org/2013/07/31/flat-abs-in-5-minutes-workout/

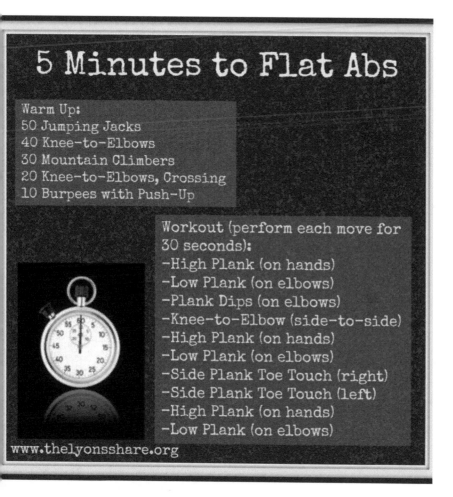

5 Minutes to Flat Abs

Warm Up:
50 Jumping Jacks
40 Knee-to-Elbows
30 Mountain Climbers
20 Knee-to-Elbows, Crossing
10 Burpees with Push-Up

Workout (perform each move for 30 seconds):
-High Plank (on hands)
-Low Plank (on elbows)
-Plank Dips (on elbows)
-Knee-to-Elbow (side-to-side)
-High Plank (on hands)
-Low Plank (on elbows)
-Side Plank Toe Touch (right)
-Side Plank Toe Touch (left)
-High Plank (on hands)
-Low Plank (on elbows)

www.thelyonsshare.org

For a 25-minute full-body and cardio workout, try this **5-4-3-2-1 Blast-Off workout.**

Find full descriptions at:

www.thelyonsshare.org/2014/01/29/5-4-3-2-1-blast-off-workout/ or Google "Lyons Share 5-4-3-2-1 workout" and click on the first result.

blast off
5-4-3-2-1 ^ Workout

5 5 backwards lunges (L), 1 hop — **x5**

4 Walk out to plank, 5 plank jacks, 1 push-up, walk up to standing — **x5**

3 5 backwards lunges (R), 1 hop — **x5**

2 5 bicep curls, 1 overhead press — **x5**

1 5 squats, 1 hop — **x5**

Repeat entire workout 5 times!

www.TheLyonsShare.org

If you have weights handy, try this **Arm and Ab Power Circuit Workout.**

Find full descriptions at:

www.thelyonsshare.org/2013/11/06/arm-and-ab-power-circuit-workout/, or Google "Lyons Share Arm and Ab Power Circuit" and click on the first result.

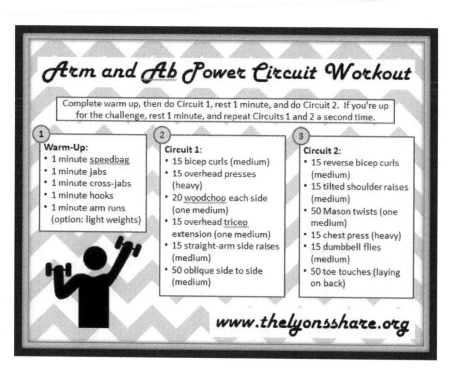

Arm and Ab Power Circuit Workout

Complete warm up, then do Circuit 1, rest 1 minute, and do Circuit 2. If you're up for the challenge, rest 1 minute, and repeat Circuits 1 and 2 a second time.

1 Warm-Up:
- 1 minute speedbag
- 1 minute jabs
- 1 minute cross-jabs
- 1 minute hooks
- 1 minute arm runs (option: light weights)

2 Circuit 1:
- 15 bicep curls (medium)
- 15 overhead presses (heavy)
- 20 woodchop each side (one medium)
- 15 overhead tricep extension (one medium)
- 15 straight-arm side raises (medium)
- 50 oblique side to side (medium)

3 Circuit 2:
- 15 reverse bicep curls (medium)
- 15 tilted shoulder raises (medium)
- 50 Mason twists (one medium)
- 15 chest press (heavy)
- 15 dumbbell flies (medium)
- 50 toe touches (laying on back)

www.thelyonsshare.org

For another arms and abs focused workout, try this **Burnin' Arms and Abs Circuit.**

Find full descriptions at:

www.thelyonsshare.org/2013/10/08/burnin-arms-and-abs-circuit-workout/, or Google "Lyons Share Burnin Arms and Abs" and click on the first result.

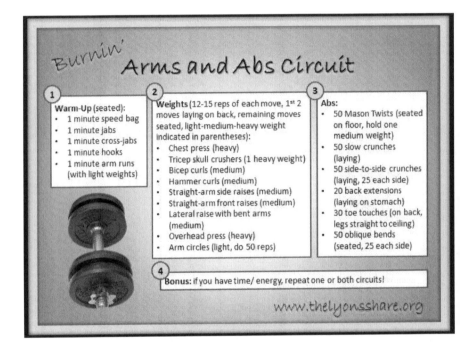

Burnin' Arms and Abs Circuit

1

Warm-Up (seated):
- 1 minute speed bag
- 1 minute jabs
- 1 minute cross-jabs
- 1 minute hooks
- 1 minute arm runs (with light weights)

2

Weights (12-15 reps of each move, 1st 2 moves laying on back, remaining moves seated, light-medium-heavy weight indicated in parentheses):
- Chest press (heavy)
- Tricep skull crushers (1 heavy weight)
- Bicep curls (medium)
- Hammer curls (medium)
- Straight-arm side raises (medium)
- Straight-arm front raises (medium)
- Lateral raise with bent arms (medium)
- Overhead press (heavy)
- Arm circles (light, do 50 reps)

3

Abs:
- 50 Mason Twists (seated on floor, hold one medium weight)
- 50 slow crunches (laying)
- 50 side-to-side crunches (laying, 25 each side)
- 20 back extensions (laying on stomach)
- 30 toe touches (on back, legs straight to ceiling)
- 50 oblique bends (seated, 25 each side)

4

Bonus: if you have time/ energy, repeat one or both circuits!

www.thelyonsshare.org

If you're feeling patriotic, try this **9/11 Memorial** workout, which can be done in about 20 minutes.

For full descriptions, visit:

www.thelyonsshare.org/2013/09/11/911-memorial-workout/ or Google "Lyons Share 9/11 Memorial Workout" and click on the first result.

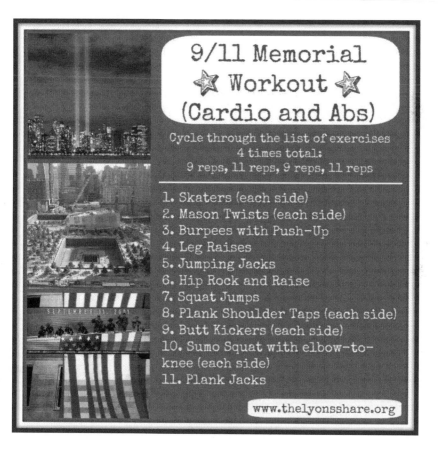

9/11 Memorial ⭐ Workout ⭐ (Cardio and Abs)

Cycle through the list of exercises 4 times total: 9 reps, 11 reps, 9 reps, 11 reps

1. Skaters (each side)
2. Mason Twists (each side)
3. Burpees with Push-Up
4. Leg Raises
5. Jumping Jacks
6. Hip Rock and Raise
7. Squat Jumps
8. Plank Shoulder Taps (each side)
9. Butt Kickers (each side)
10. Sumo Squat with elbow-to-knee (each side)
11. Plank Jacks

www.thelyonsshare.org

If you are feeling even more patriotic, try this **4th of July** workout, which can be done in 25 minutes.

For full descriptions, visit:

http://www.thelyonsshare.org/2013/07/03/4th-of-july-circuit-workout-plus-views-from-my-recent-runs/ or Google "Lyons Share 4th of July workout" and click on the first result.

4TH OF JULY 7/4/13 WORKOUT

13 moves, 7 reps per move. Repeat entire circuit 4 times (30 second rest break between each circuit)

1. Burpees (with push-up)
2. Squats
3. Star jumps
4. Forward lunge (13 each leg)
5. V-ups
6. Push-ups
7. Tuck jumps
8. Oblique dips (13 each side)
9. Chair step-ups (13 each side)
10. Jumping jacks
11. Tricep dips
12. Skater lunges (13 each side)
13. Mason twists (13 each side)

*Bonus: on last round, do 70 mason twists!

WWW.THELYONSSHARE.ORG

For a 10-minute, abdominal-focused workout, try this **ab burner.**

Find full descriptions at http://www.thelyonsshare.org/2014/03/19/ you-get-what-you-work-for-10-minute-ab-burner/ or Google "Lyons Share ab burner" and click on the first result.

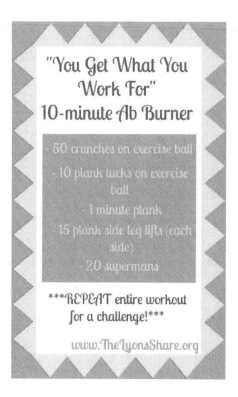

"You Get What You Work For"
10-minute Ab Burner

- 50 crunches on exercise ball
- 10 plank tucks on exercise ball
- 1 minute plank
- 15 plank side leg lifts (each side)
- 20 supermans

REPEAT entire workout for a challenge!

www.TheLyonsShare.org

If you're in a hotel or have access to a treadmill, try this **ABCBC Treadmill** workout.

For full descriptions, visit:

www.thelyonsshare.org/2013/08/21/calorie-blasting-abcbc-treadmill-workout/ or Google "Lyons Share ABCBC Workout" and click on the first result.

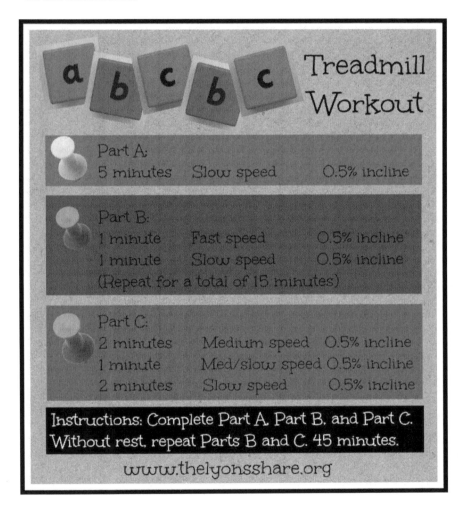

Chapter Six

Making it Work

Overview

By this point, I hope you're convinced that drinking more water, eating more vegetables, and reducing your added sugar intake would all benefit your health greatly. When all is said and done, though, none of the information in the book is valuable if you can't implement it. So if any part of it feels overwhelming, take a step back and think how you can take what you've learned and apply it to your own life. Maybe you can't make a veggie pack for every day, but you can commit to ordering a side salad every time you eat at a restaurant. Maybe you're not willing to eliminate your daily Starbucks run, but you can order plain coffee with stevia and milk instead of your usual Frappuccino every other day. These are all great changes! Remember, it's about progress, not about perfection.

In this chapter, I'll discuss several of the most common scenarios that make it tough to stick to your health goals: Eating at restaurants, going on vacation, traveling for work, taking a road trip, throwing together meals at the last minute, and generally living a busy life.

Eating at Restaurants: The BDD Rule

Aside from using extra fat, sugar, and salt to make food taste more appealing, restaurants often increase portion sizes so you end up eating more than you would at home. Some sources show that restaurant portions contain up to 50 percent more calories, fat, and sodium than an equivalent home-cooked meal.[75] Unfortunately, we don't reduce our intake later in the day to make up for this extra. One study showed that teenagers ate, on average, 309 more calories on days that they ate at fast-food restaurants (and 267 more calories on days that they ate at full-service restaurants).[76] When we dine at home, we don't have the bread-basket, the appetizer course, the dessert menu, and the full bar to steer us away from healthy eating, and the huge number of choices can skew us toward less-healthy options than we would choose to make at home. Yes, eating at restaurants healthily can be hard!

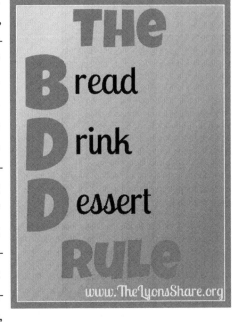

One simple tip I share with my clients to help them stay healthy even when dining out is called the "BDD rule."

On normal dinners out, I ask them to choose one option between Bread (including the breadbasket, chips, pasta, or bread as part of the meal), Drink (alcoholic or sweetened), and Dessert. On special occasions, they can choose two. And on those very special, once-in-a-blue-moon events (like a honeymoon, a restaurant they've been dying to try, or a friend's wedding), they can choose all three.

Framing it so that they get to choose one (or two, or three) of the options (rather than having to limit themselves) makes them feel more free and in control of their choices, and doesn't seem so oppressive.

Most of the time, the bread basket just doesn't look that great to me, and it's not hard to pass up. But if I didn't have the BDD rule in mind, I might mindlessly chomp on a few pieces of bread to pass the time until my meal came. Using the BDD rule is one of the many tricks I use (on myself and my clients) to help keep restaurant meals as healthy as possible. The BDD Rule prevents us from piling on the unnecessary calories and ensures that we leave feeling energized and satisfied, rather than weighed down and regretful.

Going on Vacation

When my clients have been making so much progress in their health and have vacation plans in the future, they tend to panic. What will happen to their dedication to healthy eating? Will they re-gain the 30 pounds they've lost during their 5-day vacation? Will they completely forget how to eat and live healthily, and go terribly off track? Will they be completely miserable the entire time, having to forego the famous crepes in France or their grandmother's delicious casserole?

These statements might seem silly right now, but I assure you that people do feel as if all their hard work will go down the drain when they go on vacation. When I tell them my personal philosophy on keeping up healthy habits while on vacation, they're often surprised by how simple it seems.

You see, health is about consistency ... about the choices we make day-in and day-out, month after month and year after year.

Skipping one workout or eating one unhealthy meal isn't going to ruin anything. If you are diligent in keeping up your healthy habits for the 95 percent of the year that you're not on vacation, I think you should relax your limitations and not worry so much about health while on vacation.

My vacation philosophy is this: Stick to what makes you feel great, but don't skimp on enjoying the special treats that make vacation feel indulgent. If you'll look back and regret not eating something, then eat it! The opportunities to enjoy traditional cuisine, special treats, and family traditions don't come around very often. If you will regret not getting enough sleep on vacation because you wanted to be sure to get in your workout before the kids woke up, then sleep in! You have 51 weeks of the year to encourage yourself to wake up early and fit in that workout.

There are some healthy habits that I keep up even while on vacation, because they make me feel my best. If these seem overly strict or imposing to you, you may choose to keep up other healthy habits and ignore these. But these habits make me feel my best, so I see no reason to forego them on vacation!

Healthy hydration is my favorite health habit to keep up, even while on vacation. As I mentioned, I get a headache whenever I'm dehydrated, which is something I don't want to deal with on vacation. I'm more likely to be drinking alcohol on vacation, as well, so I have extra risk of being dehydrated. For this reason, I'm sure to always keep my water with me, even on vacation, and even if that means having to find a convenience store to stock up on water bottles.

Exercising makes me feel energized, happy, and relaxed, so I'm sure to include it in some form every day, even on vacation. My vacation exercise might be a hike, a walk, or a day on the ski slopes instead of a run, but I still get in something. Touring a new city by foot not only makes me feel better than taking a taxi everywhere, it also gives me a better feel for the city's culture, people, and layout.

While it's sometimes hard to get in as many vegetables on vacation as I would at home, I do my best to include them whenever I can. Going from a very high vegetable intake to almost zero will make me feel lethargic and could cause constipation or other digestive issues. So, even if I don't have my regular green smoothies or roasted vegetables, I prioritize finding vegetables that I can add in to my vacation routine. I also travel with greens supplements to be sure my energy levels stay elevated!

While I'm keeping up my water and vegetable intake and exercising daily, I'm also loosening the reins on some other aspects of health. I'm far more likely to indulge in dessert on vacation, for example. I am sure to let myself enjoy any local cuisine specialties that I wouldn't be able to find elsewhere – I'd hate to miss a once-in-a-lifetime opportunity because I was worried about a few extra calories! I also may be less strict about having a balance of macronutrients or stopping myself when I'm just pleasantly full.

But I don't throw in the towel completely. I pick those things that I'll truly appreciate, and enjoy them without regret. I know my preferences, and I would always prefer to enjoy dessert rather than noshing through the breadbasket, so I'm likely to still pass on bread, even though it is vacation. And I certainly don't aim to order the least healthy thing on the menu just because "I can" while on vacation. It's all about balance, even on vacation.

In the end, do your best to maintain the healthy habits that make you feel your best, and then give yourself a break! I believe that vacation should be about enjoying your new surroundings, spending time with your family and friends, and relaxing.

If adhering to your healthy habits is going to stress you out or reduce your enjoyment, then I give you full permission to relax them while you're on vacation.

Traveling for Work

If your job is reviewing the dreamiest beach resorts or flying all over the world to observe different cultures and explore different cities, then the rest of us reading this are jealous. If you're like most people, though, traveling for work looks slightly different than traveling for vacation.

Before I became a full-time health coach, I traveled Monday through Thursday, every single week, for my management consulting job. In that role, I had to find ways to fit my healthy lifestyle into a life in conference rooms, airplanes, and hotel rooms. Being healthy on the road is difficult, for sure, but it *is* possible ... and it's also worth it.

While you're traveling for work, do your best to plan in advance. If you know you'll be heading to a client dinner, check out the menu online and identify the options that will make you feel best and meet your health goals. If you know you'll be driving in your car on sales calls, hit the grocery store briefly to load up on portable car snacks that will prevent you from hitting the drive-through.

Don't let the change in routine take you away from your routine healthy habits, like drinking plenty of water and fitting in some exercise. Be sure to bring a refillable water bottle on your trip, and carry it with you just as you would if you were at home. If you commit yourself to maintaining your workout schedule despite being on the road, it is absolutely possible!

Preparing Travel Snacks

Before you even leave on your trip, be sure to load up on healthy snacks for your travel bag. I like to head to the airport armed with several of the following options, to ensure that I have healthy options when hunger strikes, even if the airport food options are limited.

- **CUT-UP RAW VEGGIES.** Most veggies will be just fine unrefrigerated for a few hours. For some extra flavor, look for individual cups of guacamole or hummus (less than 3 ounces each, so they go through security), or grab some mustard or salsa from a restaurant in the airport. I used to bring leftover roasted vegetables on planes, but their off-putting smell travels quickly on planes, so I recommend sticking with raw veggies.

- **FRUIT.** Go for fruit that isn't super hard to eat and holds up reasonably well with a few bumps in your carry-on bag. I like grapes, cherries, apples, oranges, and nectarines for traveling.

- **PROTEIN/ENERGY BARS.** As always, I'd prefer to get my protein from whole food sources, but that can be tough to do on the road. I love Larabars, KIND bars, Vega bars, Quest bars, or Tanka beef jerky bars.

- **"CHIP IMPOSTORS."** If you find yourself craving something salty, it can be hard to pass up that giant bag of chips you see at the newsstand. Instead, pack some bean snacks (Enlightened makes tasty, crunchy versions), a single-serving bag of Popchips, a package of seaweed snacks (Annie Chun's, SeaSnax, or Gimme have good options), or some freeze-dried fruits or veggies. They're a great way to satisfy your cravings for crunch in a healthy way!

- **NUTS/ TRAIL MIX/ NUT BUTTER.** I love traveling with 100-calorie bags of almonds (natural, dry roasted, or cocoa flavored are my favorite!), or individual portions of trail mix without much added sugar. I know from experience that it's tough for me to limit my portions when I'm eating out of a big bag of trail mix (and even healthy snacks should be eaten in moderation!), so I try to stick to single-serving packages. I also bring single-serve packets of nut butter to squeeze onto fruit/ celery for some healthy fats, or just eat straight up in an "emergency"! I love 90-calorie packets of Barney Butter, or Justin's maple almond butter for a special treat!

- **PROTEIN SNACKS.** It is hard to find portable protein options, but I often carry protein powders that can be mixed with water (I like Only Protein or Amazing Meal), string cheese, or hard-boiled eggs.

- **WATER!** If you do nothing else while you travel, please drink a ton of water! Flying is very dehydrating, and we can often mistake thirst for hunger. I drank a full liter on each of my two recent flights, and still felt the need to chug a liter on my drive into town. If you don't want to pay an arm and a leg, bring an empty bottle through security and fill it up at the water fountains. Whatever it takes, just drink!

Exercising while Traveling

It's hard to stick to your normal exercise routine while traveling, but it's still possible to fit in some movement. Here are a few tips to help you maintain fitness on the road:

1. **RUN (OR WALK!) LOCALLY.** One of the reasons I used to enjoy traveling for work was that I got to run in new locations all the time. As long as you scope out safe areas, and take appropriate safety precautions (run in daylight if you can, or wear reflective/lighted clothing; always preview the area via online maps, or search for other runners' routes via MapMyRun or GoogleMaps; wear a RoadID or carry an ID with you), I think

running in new areas is a fun way to explore a new location and keep your workouts exciting! There are many local running groups that accept visitors, so if you prefer running in groups, do a quick Google search for the area you are visiting.

2. **WORK OUT EARLY.** I know, I know – it is often painful to roll out of bed at zero-dark-thirty! But this is often the only way to guarantee that your workout will happen on a busy work day, so try to stick to morning workouts as much as possible.

3. **MIX IT UP.** Even on the busiest of travel days, it's often possible to squeeze in 10-15 minute bursts of interval or strength training, straight from your hotel room. You can use the ones I mentioned in Chapter 5, make up your own, or head to Pinterest for inspiration (follow The Lyons' Share "workouts" board for hundreds of do-anywhere workouts!).

4. **KEEP IT SHORT ON BUSY DAYS.** We all have those days where every precious second counts, but even on those days, *something* is a whole lot better than nothing! Try to squeeze in whatever you can, even on busy weeks – you'll have more energy and feel more accomplished afterward.

5. **GET RUNNING ROUTES FROM YOUR HOTEL.** Westin chains offer index card-sized printouts of local running routes, and many other hotel chains will be able to point you in the right direction, if you don't feel like exploring yourself!

6. **PLAN YOUR ACCOMMODATIONS AT HOTEL CHAINS THAT OFFER FITNESS CENTERS.** Even though I prefer running outside, there's always that time when I'm completely time-squeezed, the weather is awful, or I need to have my phone right at hand. In those instances, having a hotel gym is

invaluable. I always try to check the website before making my reservation to ensure that a gym will be available.

7. **TRAVEL COMFORTABLY.** Walk as much as possible while traveling – in the airports, while commuting, or anywhere else you can! Walking is a great way to squeeze in exercise without thinking about it or taking time away from your trip. If I have a few minutes to kill in an airport, I'll usually try to walk up and down the hallways rather than sitting, just to get in a bit of movement.

8. **GO UP.** Hotel staircases provide a great workout when you're tight on time or don't want to run or hit the gym. Plus, you get to feel hard-core if someone enters the staircase and you're hammering out stair sprints!

9. **MAINTAIN MUSCLE AND JOINT HEALTH.** For some reason, traveling tends to make our other healthy habits fall by the wayside. So, make sure to stretch, ice, and rest just as you would while at home. Taking care of your muscles and joints pays off multiples in the long run!

Road Trips

If you're heading out on a long road trip, it can be hard to resist the McDonald's, Dairy Queen, or Sonic drive-throughs that seem to pop up at every corner. It's even more important to start your trip armed with healthy snacks (like the ones mentioned on previous pages), so that you never get so hungry that you're forced to make choices you otherwise wouldn't. The few minutes of preparation that it takes to load up a cooler with healthy options will pay off in leaps and bounds when you arrive at your destination feeling energized and healthy.

Of course, part of the reason we often finish a day of driving feeling like we could sleep for hours is that we've been so sedentary the entire time. In my mind, a long road trip is not an excuse to forego any exercise!

Here are seven ways to fit in exercise during a road trip:

1. **EXERCISE BEFORE YOU LEAVE.** Yes, it can seem difficult to wake up early to fit in a workout when you'll be spending a long, tiring day at the wheel. However, it will give you *more* energy to complete your drive safely, not to mention improve your health. Just get it in!

2. **MOVE AROUND (SAFELY) WHILE DRIVING.** A quick Google search will show some simple road trip stretches that you can incorporate into your drive. In addition, I try to remember to shift around in my seat, just to make sure I'm not sitting too still for too long.

3. **AT STOP LIGHTS,** take the opportunity to (quickly) put the car in park, lift your foot up and roll your ankle, roll your neck, and other things you may not be able to do while driving.

4. **EACH TIME YOU STOP FOR GAS,** food, or to use the restroom, make a few laps around the parking lot or do 100 jumping jacks. It may seem silly, but you'll likely never see those people again, and the movement adds up! On one particularly long day of driving, I wound up with 1,300 jumping jacks!

5. **EACH TIME YOU STOP,** take a few minutes to stretch! Your hip flexors can get especially tight while driving, so always make sure to stretch them when you stand up from the car.

6. **DRINK A LOT OF WATER!** This will make frequent stops more necessary, and will help you fit in #4 and #5 more frequently!

7. **RIGHT BEFORE EACH MEAL, DO A MINI-BOOTCAMP.** Of course, you don't want to be dripping sweat for the rest of your ride, but if you do a quick 5 minutes of jumping jacks, squats, lunges, and some walking, you should reap the benefits of a bit of movement without wearing yourself out.

Throwing Together Meals: The MVP Rule

Do you ever find yourself peering into the refrigerator at 7 p.m., already hungry, and just unable to figure out what to make for dinner? You want to prepare something healthy, but you don't have time, energy, or patience to cook an elaborate meal, and you just can't think of anything else healthy. I've been there, too! (Incidentally, way back in 2011, over 10 million searches *per day* were done for recipes.[77] and I'd imagine the growth since then is stunning!)

To help my clients out on their busiest nights, I came up with three easy tips to pull together a healthy, quick, and balanced meal using whatever you have in your refrigerator and pantry. Introducing ... the MVP Rule!

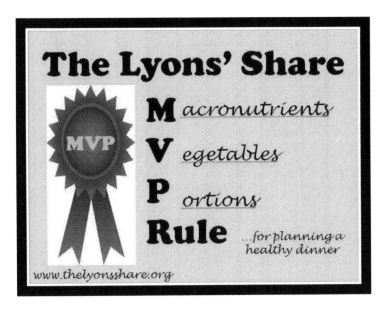

By focusing on Macronutrients, Vegetables, and Portions, you can ensure you have a healthy dinner – whether you spend hours putting it together, or throw it together at the last minute!

MACRONUTRIENTS: When putting together a healthy meal, it is helpful to understand the basics of macronutrients. Don't worry, we won't get into too much detail here! The three macronutrients are carbohydrates, fats, and proteins, and they're called macronutrients because they're the nutrients your body needs in the largest quantities (micronutrients, on the other hand, are vitamins/minerals, and are needed in far smaller quantities). Simply put, macronutrients provide the calories and building blocks your body needs to function, and you need a balance of all three macronutrients to thrive. I'll be brief, but let me describe why you need each macronutrient:

- **CARBOHYDRATES:** provide energy to your body, muscles, and brain. Your body needs carbohydrates, and while limiting them works for some people, there's no reason to avoid them completely as several "fad diets" would have you do. It is healthier, though, to focus on unrefined, natural forms of carbohydrates, and to look for whole grains over white, processed grains. Fibrous foods are also a source of carbs, and your body loves fiber for healthy digestion, weight control, blood sugar control, and disease prevention!

- **FAT:** do not be afraid of fat, please! Not only is fat the most satiating macronutrient (meaning that it helps you stay full), but it is also the most efficient energy-providing macronutrient, and is necessary for many, many of your body's critical functions (like vitamin absorption, growth and development, and cell function).

- **PROTEIN:** critical for your body's growth, muscle/tissue repair, and muscle mass preservation, protein is a healthy eater's dream. It helps a meal feel substantial, keeps you full and energized, and powers your body as it gets stronger and faster!

How do you ensure a macronutrient balance in a quick meal? Make sure you get a balance of macronutrients, and look for each one of them in every meal. Good sources of carbohydrates are fruits, vegetables, and whole grains ... so toss in whatever veggies you have in your fridge, add some quinoa or brown rice, or serve squash or sweet potatoes on the side. Good sources of healthy fats are nuts, seeds (like sunflower, chia, or flax), avocados, olives, oils, and fattier fish ... so add one as an accent to your meal. Good sources of protein are chicken, fish, meats, tofu (in limited quantities), tempeh, beans, dairy (like Greek yogurt or milk), and eggs ... so make sure your meal includes at least one of these.

VEGETABLES: As we discussed in Chapter Three, vegetables are not only chock-full of disease-fighting antioxidants, but they're filling, high in fiber, and delicious.

How do you ensure you're getting plenty of vegetables in a quick meal? Simple ... pile them on! Don't fall into the trap of thinking you have a small portion of corn, potato, or other starchy vegetable on your plate, so your "vegetable" box is checked. Instead, look for a variety of colors and flavors, and include as many as you can! Return to Chapter Three for more guidance on incorporating vegetables.

PORTIONS: So many people who think they're eating the healthiest diets but are struggling to lose weight are just poorly estimating their portion sizes! It's hard to give guidelines for this one, because it's entirely dependent on each individual – how active they are, what gender/age/weight they are, how their body uniquely metabolizes food and what kind of diet works for them. Suffice it to say, for here, that being mindful of your portion sizes is a great first step!

How do you ensure you're monitoring portion sizes in a quick meal? Be reasonable about the portion sizes that you need for your activity level and goals. Work on eating mindfully, focusing on the food you're eating, and being honest with yourself. If you struggle with portion sizes, reduce your plate size – in a study published by Cornell, people served in larger bowls ate 16 percent more than those who ate out of smaller bowls, and underestimated their consumption by 7 percent more than the smaller bowl group![78]

Making Healthy Meals Fit Into Your Busy Life: Meal Planning and Food Prep

One of the most valuable lessons I share with my clients is the importance of dedicating a few hours each week to meal planning and food preparation. In today's busy world, it can be very hard to set aside a few precious hours of the weekend, and I understand that this is not a small thing to ask. But what would you say if I told you that the two or three hours you spend in meal prep on the weekend could save you four to six hours during the week ... *plus* eliminate the stress and anxiety you have over figuring out what to eat each meal during the week?

I'm sure you know the feeling – you're driving home from a meeting, ready to gnaw your arm off. It's 8 p.m. and you're debating between throwing in the towel on your health goals by driving through a fast-food window, taking another hour to prepare something healthy (did that broccoli already go bad, or could you squeeze out one more day?), and having yet another bowl of cereal. Just thinking about the decision is enough to stress you out. If you have kids, add the never-ending chorus of "Mooommmm, what's for dinner?" to the mix, and your anxiety levels are likely off the charts. But if you had committed two to three hours to food prep over the weekend, you wouldn't have to deal with any of this. Wouldn't that be worth the time investment?

To give a "formula" for food prep that would apply to every single reader would be next to impossible, because each person's needs vary so dramatically. How large is your family? How many meals do you eat at work, and do you have a refrigerator to store food while you are there? Do you need to rely on cold meals, or do you have a stove or microwave to heat meals up on the go? Do you go out for date night every Friday? When do you work out, and how do your post-workout fueling needs impact your meal plan? Does little Timmy hate spinach and Sally loves broccoli? Do you like to go grocery shopping once a week at a large commercial grocery store, or twice weekly at a small co-op? These are just some of the many questions that I ask my clients as I help them develop a plan for their weekly food preparation, and a few of the questions you need to ask yourself before beginning this helpful habit.

The first, and most important, step of building in this habit is to block aside time on your calendar weekly. Like any habit, it is far less likely to actually happen if it's not given its spot on our agenda. To get the official Lyons' Share meal planning template, download the *Start Here* free bonuses at **www.StartHereBonus.com.**

Second, choose two things that you want to prepare during the first week. You'll have plenty of time to prepare more and more as you get more adept with your food prep, but for this week, just choose two things.

Third, actually do it! Put on some music or a podcast to make it fun, and try to minimize any other distractions. Commit to staying in the kitchen until your preparation is done. I like having a written plan or a list of what I'm going to prepare, and then I get all of my ingredients, recipes, cutting boards, and tools out and ready before I begin. Chefs call this technique "mise en place," which means "putting in place."

Finally, once you're done preparing, package everything up in glass containers or Tupperwares. You want to have easy access to the meals you've prepared during the week, to ensure that you actually use the fruits of your labor!

If you have kids, I highly recommend posting a meal list at the beginning of each week. My clients who post a meal list are so grateful to not have to deal with the nagging daily (or hourly!) questions. Not only can the questions get old after a while, but if you don't yet know what you'll be preparing for dinner, they can also stress you out! Once you have a posted meal list, you can simply tell your child to "look at the menu" and go on with your life. The kids look forward to it, too!

So, what will you prepare for your first week? Remember, start slowly. Choose only two things to prepare this week, and build on them as you become more comfortable. Here are a few recommendations:

Breakfast
- Grab-and-Go Egg Muffins, Chapter 3

- Zucchini Apple Breakfast Muffins, Chapter 4

- Oatmeal (yes, you can prepare it in advance, then just heat it up, and add some berries, chia seeds, and a bit of honey or maple syrup when you're ready to serve!)

- Fruit (cut into bite-sized pieces, and drizzled with lemon juice to prevent browning)

- Greek yogurt mixed with chia seeds, canned pure pumpkin, cinnamon, and a few drops of stevia

Lunch/Dinner:
- Salads (keep the dressing and any moisture-heavy toppings on the side until ready to serve)

- Healthy 10-Minute Tortilla Soup, Chapter 3

- Any other crockpot chili, soup, or stew

- Chop vegetables for stir-fries and other dishes

- Bake chicken breasts for meals, sandwiches, salads

- Prepare grains (such as quinoa or brown rice) to have on hand

- Bake sweet potatoes to add to meals

- Roast vegetables to add to meals, Chapter 3

Snacks:

- Veggie packs, end of this chapter

- Fruit (cut into bite-sized pieces)

- Homemade energy balls or granola bars

- Nuts, seeds, or trail mix, portioned into individual servings

Which two items will you prepare this week?

~ Recipe: My #1 Secret to Fitting in Vegetables ~

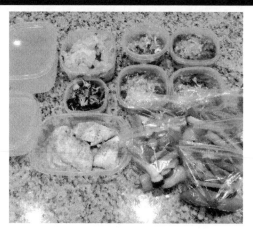

(The photo shows a typical day of Sunday food prep, including my veggie packs, roasted vegetables, baked chicken breasts, a crockpot soup, and some bone broth!)

When we have vegetables and fruits available, we are far more likely to choose them. If we have vegetable sticks ready to go when we're running out the door, we're much more likely to resist visiting a fast-food drive-through or grabbing a gas station snack, because we've filled up on delicious vegetables!

I enjoy raw vegetables as an afternoon snack almost every single day, but I don't have time to cut them and prepare them every day. So, each Sunday, I make what I call "veggie packs." I gather and chop whatever raw vegetables looked great at the Farmer's Market or grocery store – see the list below for some of my favorites!. I take out 5-7 Ziploc bags or small Tupperware containers, and I divide the cut vegetables into each container. Then, I have a pre-made snack for every day of the week, and can ensure I'm getting in a few good servings, even on the busiest of days. If I want a bit more flavor for my veggie pack, I'll sometimes spray in a bit of olive oil and sea salt, or dip my vegetables in hummus or salsa.

I challenge you to try veggie packs this week – I'll bet you'll be grateful to have the preparation taken care of, and to have healthy snacks available to you!

~ Recipe: Veggie Packs ~

You know that getting in your vegetables is important, and it's also difficult on those days when you're on the run. It's easy to resort to packaged and refined snack foods like energy bars, chips, or cookies when we don't plan in advance. By spending 10 minutes preparing veggie packs on Sunday afternoons, though, you ensure that you'll have a nutrient-dense snack every single day!

Make 5 veggie packs each Sunday, and force yourself to grab a pack every day of the week as you head out the door. You'll be amazed at how easy it is to get in this extra serving of vegetables when it's prepared and ready to go!

INGREDIENTS

5-10 cups of raw vegetables, including:

- Cherry tomatoes
- Celery
- Baby carrots, or whole carrots, sliced
- Jicama
- Snap peas
- Snow peas
- Mini bell peppers, or sliced bell peppers
- Sliced cucumbers (the small Persian cucumbers are especially delicious!)
- Broccoli
- Cauliflower

OPTIONAL TOPPINGS

- Olive oil spray and sea salt (spray on each morning; if you add the oil on Sunday, your veggies will be soggy by Friday or before)
- Individual packets of hummus, salsa, mustard, or light dressing

You'll need 5 portable containers (Tupperware containers, mason jars, or Ziploc baggies)

INSTRUCTIONS

- Divide vegetables evenly into 5 containers. Do not seal all the way – a bit of air helps keep the veggies crisp!
- Store in refrigerator, and grab one every day!

CHAPTER SEVEN

CULTIVATE GRATITUDE AND SELF-FORGIVENESS

A Daily Attitude of Gratitude

*H*ow often do you pause in the middle of the day, take a deep breath, and realize how grateful you are for those big things in your life – your health, your family, your freedom, your safety? How often do you pause in the midst of enjoying a nice meal and reflect on your gratitude for the nourishing food on your plate? How often do you make a point to really *feel* gratitude?

If you're like most people, the answer probably is "not very often." Aside from Thanksgiving Day, we are accustomed to going through our lives without consciously expressing our gratitude for the things we have, the emotions we feel, or the situations and relationships that we've created for ourselves. We're simply too busy to pause and reflect on our gratitude. If asked whether or not we are grateful for our families, of course, the vast majority of us would answer that we are. But we still go through days, weeks, and even years without pausing to recognize that feeling.

The word "gratitude" is becoming increasingly popular in health circles these days, and for good reason. In fact, practicing gratitude daily not only makes you feel happier and more appreciative, it also has a huge beneficial impact on your overall health!

Studies link gratitude to reduced stress, reduced addictive tendencies, decreased depression, improved sleep quality, and better overall physical health. Those who practice gratitude have better mental health, and are consequently more likely to choose healthy activities and seek medical help when needed.[79] One study even shows a 76 percent improvement in body image by those who practice gratitude![80]

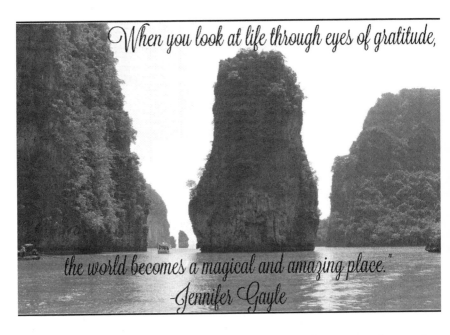

When you look at life through eyes of gratitude, the world becomes a magical and amazing place."
-Jennifer Gayle

Aside from the incredible health benefits, going about your day-to-day life with an attitude of gratitude makes everything seem easier and more harmonious. You've been there, right? Sometimes you'll have a day where you wake up with a smile, and things just seem to go "your way." Even when something doesn't go quite your way, you take it in stride, because it just *feels* like an amazing day! Of course, there are also those days when you grudgingly roll out of bed with a bad attitude, and it seems like *nothing* in your life is right. Your lack of gratitude casts a dark gray cloud over every single aspect of your life. It's pretty amazing what a difference your attitude of gratitude can make!

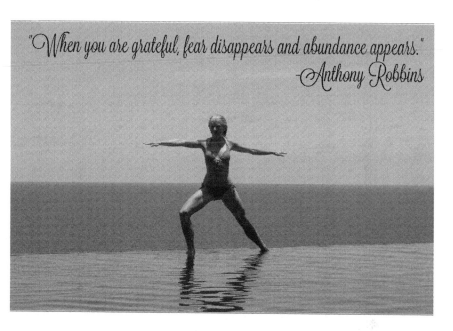

"When you are grateful, fear disappears and abundance appears."
—Anthony Robbins

When I stop and think about it, I have so, so many things to be grateful for, and I'm guessing you do, too. Even on the worst days, I can identify many things that I feel so lucky to have … from the smallest (my morning cup of coffee or tea!) to the largest (my amazing husband, the health of my family, and the assurance that I have food to eat and a roof over my head). Without stopping to think about these things consciously, though, we often don't even realize how lucky we are, and we certainly don't get the amazing health benefits.

In order to make gratitude a part of our daily routines, we need to create a habit. Some people like to immediately think of a few things they are grateful for immediately upon waking, maybe even before getting out of bed. Some prefer to journal at the end of the day, reflecting upon things that happened during the day that made them feel grateful. Some put a virtual post-it note on their computer screen, or put a Word document on their computer desktop, and jot their gratitude list there daily. Some set a daily calendar alarm to ring on their phone or computer mid-day, as a reminder to pause and practice gratitude.

For me personally, one thing worked best: I bought a book. The book I use (called *The Gratitude Habit: a 365 Day Journal and Workbook*, by Wendy Meg Siegel, and available on Amazon or through other retailers) is quite simple, and consists of a few inspirational quotes, along with blank lines for me to journal in every single day. It's quite simple, but having a physical prompt to remind me to reflect has been a powerful way for me to practice gratitude daily. Each morning, before I open up my computer to address the dozens of requests, bills, business notes, and more that we are all confronted with daily, I take a few minutes to reflect on my own gratitude, and I find that the rest of my day goes much more smoothly after doing so. I've been journaling my gratitude lists for over two years now, and I can honestly say that my stress levels, sense of appreciation for my life, and ability to take challenges in stride all have improved because of it.

If you're ready to take your gratitude practice to the next level, I highly recommend reading *The Miracle Morning* by Hal Elrod. Hal, whose own story is incredibly inspiring, recommends a daily ritual including silence (or meditation), affirmations, visualization, exercise, reading, and scribing (or journaling). While it may at first seem excessive to build in time for each of these every single morning, the case made for the power of these habits is convincing - Oprah, Richard Branson, Tim Cook, Howard Schulz, and Jack Dorsey are among the many who are using *The Miracle Morning* to improve their daily productivity. I've been on my own *Miracle Morning* journey for approximately one year at the time of publication, and I can definitively say my days are less stressful, more joyful, and more productive when I wake up thirty minutes early to get in my own *Miracle Morning* routine.

As you incorporate the habits in this book to begin transforming your health, I encourage you to not forget about your mental health, as well. After all, if we are living in a state of depression or anxiety, feeling frustrated about the little things in life, or feeling emotionally out of balance, we can eat all the kale in the world and still not be truly healthy. So, create your own practice of gratitude, and see how that practice begins transforming your daily emotional wellness!

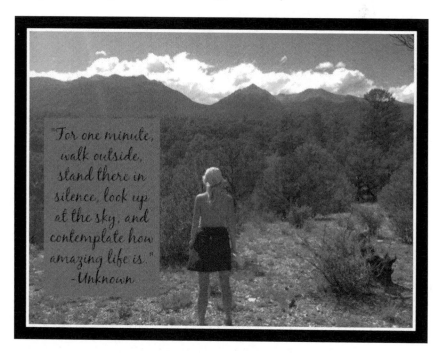

"For one minute, walk outside, stand there in silence, look up at the sky, and contemplate how amazing life is."
-Unknown

Health is an Unreachable Destination

Another aspect of mental health that I urge you to work on is being gentle with yourself. We are often our own worst critics, and it's easy to pick apart what we're doing wrong and beat ourselves up for it. Being gentle with yourself, showing gratitude daily, and striving for continuous improvement all are important ways to give yourself the respect you deserve. Let's talk about the concept of continuous improvement first.

So often, we set expectations for what our future will look like and how happy we will be after just achieving one next health goal. How many times have you said to yourself:

"I'll finally be confident once I drop these last 10 pounds"

or

"Life will be so much better if I can just get my diet under control"?

How about:

- *"I'll finally feel accomplished once I can run 5 miles straight/ bench press 100 pounds/walk 10 minutes without stopping"*

- *"I will be able to get a new job/date/opportunity once I look how I want to look"*

- *"I will allow myself to be happy/leave a dysfunctional relationship/take a vacation once I lose this pesky weight"*

If you have talked to yourself this way in the past, you're not alone. By nature, we humans don't like experiencing unpleasant emotions, and we love having a scapegoat for anything unpleasant. This helps us feel that it's not our personalities or our inner selves that are problematic, but rather an external condition.

Rather than admitting that something in our life is "wrong," we place the blame on our health. Attributing a bad situation to an external factor feels better than taking the blame ourselves. Instead of admitting that our personality wasn't a fit, it's more comfortable to rationalize a romantic rejection by thinking rejections won't happen "*10 pounds from now.*"

Not only does this not take care of the issue (we still don't have a date), but it also leaves us feeling disempowered, guilty, and ashamed. We often throw our hands up in defeat, thinking that we're just not capable of getting healthy and wondering why "everyone else" is so much healthier than we are.

We wish we had started getting healthier before, had stuck to that last diet we tried, or were able to control that late-night snacking. In this way, attributing happiness or success to one specific health milestone keeps us in a vicious cycle of depression and self-degradation.

Even worse, if we do achieve that milestone and our life is not a shining example of health and happiness, we feel as if we have failed. What happens when we lose those ten pounds and get rejected once again? Or when we finally run five miles straight and still don't feel like an athlete?

Most likely, we decide that we must have been mistaken when we set the initial goal – we probably need to lose *another* five pounds or be able to run *seven* miles straight, not just five. You can see where this cycle will lead – there is always another goal to achieve.

That brings me to the point of this section: **health is an unreachable destination.** There is no "there," no point at which medals are given out rewarding the recipient for finally achieving health, no weight or size or fitness level at which we can declare that our work is done.

I'll let you in on a little secret: Even the most famous athletes want to get a bit faster or stronger, even the highest-paid models would like to change one small thing about their bodies, and even the world's leading nutrition experts don't eat a perfect diet all the time. You don't have to place the expectation of perfection on yourself either!

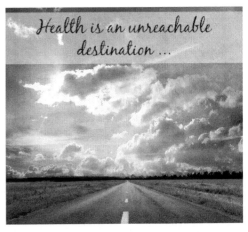

Health is an unreachable destination ...

Continuous Improvement

Instead of focusing on everything that will finally come true once your next health goal is achieved, I advise you to **strive for continuous improvement**. If your only goal each day is to be a tiny bit healthier than you were yesterday, you set yourself up for success.

From a business perspective, Toyota is a great model of continuous improvement.[81] The company teaches its employees to strive for "kaizen," a Japanese word meaning "good change," and often interpreted to mean "continuous improvement" or "self-changing for the best of all." In car manufacturing, there is always something to improve, and a constant focus on getting to the next level prevents stagnation and delinquency.

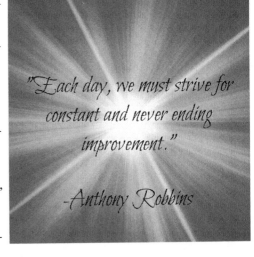

"Each day, we must strive for constant and never ending improvement."

-Anthony Robbins

Just like the car manufacturing process, our health is a perfect candidate for continuous improvement. There is always something we can make just a bit better – getting a step closer to our ideal weight, increasing the proportions of energizing and healthy foods, achieving a few extra minutes of mental clarity or another hour of sleep, or improving our fitness and physical achievements.

By looking at your health in this way, and focusing on what you can improve next rather than what is "wrong" with you at the moment, you will be better able to reduce the cycle of unfulfilled expectations. You will also prevent stagnation and achieve higher levels of health and vitality – because, after all, there is no "there," so you must constantly continue to improve!

This is not contradictory to my previous concept, of health as an unreachable destination. In both concepts, I encourage you to aim for regular, small improvements, but not to focus on a specific destination as the end-all-be-all. And, remember, never tie your feelings of self-worth to what you have or haven't achieved for your health. We are all on a journey of continuous improvement, and just by reading this book, you're well on your way.

Comparison is the Thief of Joy

Let's face it – most of us are never going to win an Olympic medal or be on the cover of the Sports Illustrated swimsuit edition, and as far as I know, there's no prize for eating the healthiest diet in the world (unless you consider a happy, vibrant, and long life a prize, which I certainly do!). Given that you're not in an actual race with anyone else, why do we find it so easy to compare ourselves to others and criticize our own bodies?

Comparison is a natural tendency for humans, but it will only leave you feeling worse about yourself. If you compare and find yourself "ahead," then you are pinning your internal thoughts about yourself to an arbitrary and meaningless target (the other person), and making yourself feel better at the expense of someone else. And, of course, if you compare and find yourself "behind," then you fail to appreciate your current successes, and feel badly about yourself for no reason.

I'm sure you've walked into a cocktail party or gym locker room and used comparison to make yourself feel better or worse. Have you thought: *"Everyone here is so thin ... they must be staring at me because I'm not a size 2"*? How about: *"Wow, she has more cellulite than I do, I must be doing great"*?

Next time you find yourself making an arbitrary comparison to your own body, I challenge you to think of a way to compliment that other person, either verbally or mentally. Turn the previous thoughts into, *"Wow, that woman smiles so brightly, she looks so confident and happy"* or *"That hairstyle is such a great compliment to her face!"* You may even smile at the person, or tell him or her the compliment out loud. It's great to lift others up when your natural tendency is to compare. Whatever you do, though, don't put yourself down when comparing yourself to others.

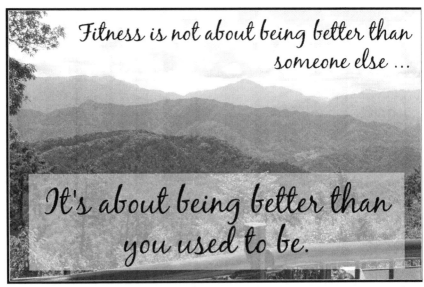

Fitness is not about being better than someone else ...

It's about being better than you used to be.

If you think you would benefit from a supportive community that encourages others' success rather than comparing in a negative manner, join the Start Here Community at **www. StartHereCommunity.com**.

Appreciating Your Current Position

As we're on the journey of continuous improvement, it is helpful to take a moment to appreciate our current health successes. Our bodies are truly remarkable machines, and too often we focus on criticizing them for the extra weight that they carry, or the pain that wasn't there yesterday.

When we take the time to reflect on our progress, though, we realize that we are continuously improving ourselves in ways that we often take for granted. It's so easy to think negative thoughts about the ways we are "failing" or "not living up to our goals/potential," and we often let those thoughts overcrowd the feelings of accomplishment.

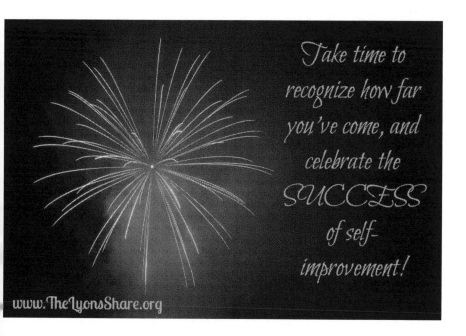

Take time to recognize how far you've come, and celebrate the SUCCESS of self-improvement!

www.TheLyonsShare.org

Right now, please mentally note a few things you are proud of accomplishing for your health. Sure, there is potential for improvement on the horizon, and once you finish this book, you're going to go headfirst after that potential. But I want to be sure you appreciate where you stand today before we begin making that progress. Have you committed to a workout routine and stuck with it? Changed from chips to apple slices in the office cafeteria? Kicked your habit of diet sodas?

Take a moment to congratulate yourself for how far you've come so far - get a manicure after work, simply recognize the accomplishment and savor the feeling of pride, or let yourself spend 5 minutes reading for pleasure after you put the kids to bed. Congratulations, I am proud of you ... now be proud of yourself, too! I'm confident you'll feel better when you appreciate yourself.

~ Recipe: An Exercise in Gratitude ~

This "recipe" will help jump-start your practice of gratitude and self-forgiveness. Set aside 10 minutes to do this in silence, without distractions!

INGREDIENTS

- An open mind
- A clean sheet of paper and a pen

INSTRUCTIONS

1. Close your eyes. Focus on your breath for 2 minutes, to center yourself and get ready to begin your practice of gratitude. As you breathe, appreciate your heart, which continues to beat every moment of every day, and your body, which carries you through every day.

2. Make a list of 20 things for which you are grateful today. Because this is your first day, just let the words flow – the items can be as simple or as grandiose as you choose. Try to get all of your feelings down on paper.

3. Reflect again. Take one more minute to close your eyes and appreciate the 20 items on your list. Does this help put your troubles into perspective?

4. Determine how you will continue your practice of gratitude daily. Will you buy a book, start a practice of making your gratitude list each morning, or put a reminder on your computer? Do you want to write one thing per day, or five? Do you want to silently think about your gratitude while lying in bed, or call up an accountability partner on the phone and tell him or her your list while you're enjoying a walk outside? Whatever works for you, start tomorrow! Just list a few things every single day, and watch how it transforms your attitude.

CHAPTER EIGHT

THE MISSING PIECE

Why It Hasn't Worked Before

I hope you've learned a lot in the previous seven chapters, and that you feel inspired to incorporate many of these changes into your own life. I intended to present the information in a useable, educational, and approachable way, and broke it down into simple steps that I have proven to be effective with my clients. I know these steps work because I've seen them work so many times.

I also know, though, that you were likely familiar with at least some of these concepts before you started reading *Start Here*. You probably already knew that vegetables were healthy, and if you really thought about it, you might have realized that you weren't drinking enough water on a daily basis.

So why do we need to keep hearing these concepts over and over again? Why do I have so much success with my clients by getting them to incorporate these small changes into their lives, when you have tried drastic measures and intense diets before, only to return to your old ways?

The missing piece is simple: We all need motivation and accountability.

We need accountability day-in and day-out, consistently, steadily, over time. Not the kind of accountability that makes you feel you have failed completely if you stray from the plan just the tiniest bit, but the kind of accountability that encourages you to stay the course and keep reaching toward your goal. The kind of accountability that motivates you to be the best you can be, and go after the goals that you set for yourself. The kind of accountability that makes you order the grilled asparagus instead of the french fries, or makes you strap on your running shoes even though it's raining, and still brings a smile to your face when you do so. We all need regular motivational reminders to inspire us to keep going, even when the going gets tough.

The Value of Daily Motivation

If your first reaction to the idea of accountability is, "I don't need someone to hold my hand every step of the way," I encourage you to think about the last time you set a goal – health or otherwise. Did you reach it? If so, you likely had a clear motivation to succeed (take, for example, a goal set out for you by your boss, with the implicit suggestion that you won't have a job if you don't reach the goal). You were probably reminded of this motivation every single day, either by yourself or someone else. That daily dose of motivation was critical to your success.

If, on the other hand, you didn't succeed, maybe you lost focus or other priorities got in the way. Unfortunately, we let this happen with our health regularly – prioritizing work, family, fun, or something else over our own health. Most of us need daily motivation and nearly constant reminders to achieve our goals, to ensure that life doesn't just "get in the way."

The need for daily motivation is OK! It doesn't make you less of a person, indicate that you have less willpower, or mean that you "failed" at motivating yourself. In fact, if you realize that daily motivation helps you maintain the behaviors you want to maintain, you will have more success with your health goals!

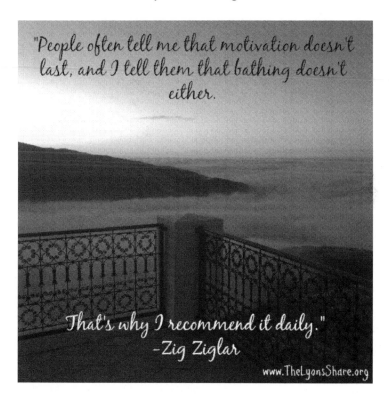

"People often tell me that motivation doesn't last, and I tell them that bathing doesn't either. That's why I recommend it daily."
—Zig Ziglar
www.TheLyonsShare.org

7 Tips to Boost Your Motivation Daily

1. **MAKE UP YOUR MIND BEFORE YOU HAVE THE CHOICE.** Making up your mind earlier makes it far more likely that you will attain the goals you set for yourself. If you set your alarm for 5:00 a.m., and tell yourself you'll wake up to work out if you feel good, there's a strong chance it's not going to happen. However, if you go to bed already *knowing* that you will wake up without snoozing and without questioning, giving yourself no choice, you're more likely to actually get it done. If you sign up for a fitness class and know you'll lose

your money if you skip, the decision has already been made, so you're more likely to actually attend.

2. **PLAN AHEAD.** Planning ahead is critical to almost every aspect of health. Do your best to fit in weekend meal prep, make healthy meals in advance (and store them in the freezer for inevitable busy nights), schedule workouts in your calendar, and decide the night before exactly which healthy behaviors you'll choose for the following day.

3. **FIND YOUR "WHY."** It's helpful to remind yourself of the reason you're doing what you're doing over and over again. Feeling good *now* (by sitting on the couch, eating that third slice of pie, etc.) will always take precedence over your long-term goals, *unless* you can remind yourself of why you want to accomplish them. Regardless of the goal, it's important to have a truly deep-seated reason for accomplishing it. Finding this why often requires some thought, self-reflection, and soul-searching ... the real why is often not something on the surface level. A *Forbes* article on this topic says, "knowing your why is an important first step in figuring out how to achieve the goals that excite you and create a life you enjoy living (versus merely surviving!)."[82]

Most of my Health Coaching clients say they "just want to get healthy" ... because they know they "should," because they're getting a bit older, or because they've gained a bit of weight. But part of my job as a Health Coach is to dig a bit deeper and find their true motivation for wanting to improve their health. For a woman who says she's getting a bit older, the why might be that her husband's health is faltering, her kids are now on their own, her best friend passed away unexpectedly, and this all leaves her feeling like she's headed for a rapid decline if she doesn't change something quickly.

For another client who says she's gained a bit of weight, the why might be that she hasn't dated in 3 years and doesn't feel good enough about herself to reflect a positive outward image to potential partners. Do you see how your true why is just a bit deeper than your initial reaction?

So, whatever your goal is, I encourage you to find your why. You can continue asking yourself why over and over in order to find the response. If you say you want to start exercising, ask *why*. If you respond that you think you "should," ask *why*. If you say because you want to be healthy, ask *why*. If you say because you want to live 50 more years, ask *why* .... you get the point. Continue this until you get to a deep-seated response that really means something to you.

4. **WRITE YOURSELF A NOTE.** Place it somewhere very visible to you, so that you see it every day. For example, I have my monthly business goals posted right next to my workstation in my office. If I'm working on something in particular during a given week for my health, I'll set calendar reminders to help me remember my specific goals (for example, "drink tea instead of eating dessert tonight!").

5. **CREATE HABITS THAT ENABLE YOUR CHOSEN BEHAVIORS.** If you want to work out in the morning, lay out your workout clothes the night before (or sleep in them). If you want to drink more water, set out a given number of water bottles each morning (or fill a pitcher in the morning and aim to empty it by the end of the day). If you want to eat more vegetables, keep them in plain sight so you're more likely to reach for them. If you want to drink less alcohol, schedule your next get-together with friends while going for a walk or checking out a new dance class, rather than sitting at a bar. If you want to start walking daily, put a post-it note on your dog's leash

to actually walk with the dog, not just stand there scrolling through your phone while he does his business. Regardless of your chosen behavior, create a habit that will make it easier for you to achieve your goals.

6. **USE SOCIAL MEDIA TO YOUR ADVANTAGE.** The instant gratification we get from seeing "likes" on our social media posts can help boost our dedication to achieving our goals, whether they be health-related or not. Simply stating your goals publicly dramatically increases your likelihood of follow-through, since you don't want to be embarrassed or proven wrong by not achieving what you stated. New research is being done to show that those who post regularly to social media not only feel more motivated, but also have more success when it comes to weight loss, BMI reduction, and waist-to-hip ratio.[83]

Of course, I'll recommend following The Lyons' Share on social media (find us at "The Lyons' Share Wellness" on Facebook, @TheLyonsShare on Twitter, @TheLyonsShare on Instagram, and @TheLyonsShare on Pinterest). We post motivational quotes and / or helpful articles every single day.

However, I've created an exciting opportunity exclusively for readers of *Start Here*. The Start Here Community on Facebook is an incredibly supportive health and wellness community, where you can post your successes, questions, challenges, and goals (you're more likely to succeed if you do!). I urge you to find an accountability partner (more on that in the coming pages) and invite them to join you on your *Start Here* journey. You can read the book together, develop goals together, and hold each other accountable right in the private Facebook group for *Start Here* readers only. To join (for free!), simply go to **www.StartHereCommunity.com**, and request to join. You'll be cheered on and supported the entire way!

7. **SURROUND YOURSELF WITH PEOPLE WHO SHARE YOUR GOALS.** It's a lot harder to exercise if none of your friends exercise, and it's a lot harder to choose the salad if every single one of your co-workers is choosing the fried chicken. So, find a mentor, a health coach, a family member, or a friend who shares your goals, and motivate each other daily! Find groups of people (like the Start Here Community at www.StartHereCommunity.com) who share similar goals, and support each other as you achieve them. Make it easier on yourself by being around those who encourage you!

Why We Need Accountability: A Scenario

Even if we feel incredibly motivated at the beginning of our journey, we still need accountability to stay consistent in our efforts. So many times, we'll get all riled up to "get healthy," and we'll buy new shoes or workout clothes, join a new gym, or go grocery shopping for healthy snacks. I'll use "Rhonda" as an example of someone who isn't able to reach her goals because of lack of accountability, and ends up on the dreaded diet roller coaster, climbing quickly toward her goals and then plunging downhill over and over again.

Rhonda sets aggressive goals, like *"I will work out for 90 minutes every single day this week! And eat as little as possible! That will help me lose 20 pounds before vacation next month!"* She wakes up on the morning of the first day, fits in her workout, and in the workout-induced endorphin rush, exclaims, *"This is amazing! I probably won't be able to walk tomorrow because I'm so sore, but I feel great! No more sweets ever! No more sleeping in! I'm in this for the long haul!"* She decides to skip breakfast (*"I feel so great, who needs breakfast?"*), has a salad for lunch, and daydreams about the next day's workout.

And then she crashes. The afternoon slump hits her hard, and her body is so out-of-whack that she feels like she needs a nap. She knows she shouldn't hit the vending machine (remember? *"No more sweets ever!"*), but she's just ... so ... tired. Just one bag of M&Ms won't hurt, she figures, so she grabs one, and feels better immediately.

Until the guilt hits. Then, she says to herself, *"Are you kidding? You can't even get through one day of the healthy plan?"* She feels so incapable that she goes ahead and orders a pizza for dinner. And tops it off with a pint of ice cream, because she's already ruined the day anyway. She stays up late thinking about what she did, and then turns off the next day's alarm, because she knows she won't get up and work out anyway. All bets are off. This "healthy living thing" kind of stinks.

Why We Need Accountability: A Response

Rhonda's situation might sound a bit dramatic, but it's something I see over and over again. There are many problems with the situation above. First, Rhonda's goals were far too aggressive. Going from no exercise to intense daily workouts and a "perfect" diet is not only too much to expect, it's also dangerous. When I set workout goals with my clients, I always encourage them to start slowly, like we discussed in Chapter 5. If you haven't worked out in a while, two 10-minute sessions a week might be plenty to start out! Easing into a goal slowly and gradually prevents burnout.

Second, Rhonda's goal of eating as little as possible was misguided and not specific enough to be successful. As you have learned over the previous chapters, there is no need to eat *less* food overall if you're eating the *right* foods. By trying to skip meals or limit food as much as possible, Rhonda set herself up to crave for unhealthy foods later in the day, or binge on anything she could get her hands on because she was so hungry. When I set food goals with my clients, I again encourage them to start slowly. Maybe they aim to include three fruits and vegetables each day for the first week, without restrictions on other food intake, so they don't feel deprived. Maybe they work on incorporating two specific healthy snacks into their afternoons, so they avoid the vending machine. Each goal is specific and attainable.

Third, Rhonda did not incorporate any of the tips mentioned so far. She did not have a deep-seated "why," did not create habits that enabled the behaviors she wanted to incorporate, and did not have a (virtual or in-person) support system to help her reach her goals.

Fourth, and most importantly, Rhonda was not accountable to anyone but herself. She set aggressive goals in her own mind, but didn't tell anyone about the goals and didn't have anyone to "catch" her when she began to slip up. Imagine if she had someone sending her a text message in the afternoon to check in ... do you think she would have chosen the M&Ms then? Probably not!

While we can convince ourselves to do just about anything once, we really need an accountability partner to keep us on track over the long run. It's simply too tempting to change our minds, deviate from the plan, or even throw in the towel altogether if no one is checking up on us.

The results of having someone check in with you on your progress are dramatic! A study by Stanford University found that receiving a check-in call to ask about exercise progress every two weeks increased the amount of exercise participants did by 78 percent on average.[84] Wouldn't you be more likely to get in your workout if you knew someone was going to check in on you later in the day? It's very easy to talk ourselves out of a workout in our own minds, but not so easy when we feel that we're going to disappoint someone else.

Who Will You Choose to Hold You Accountable?

Regardless of where you are on your health journey, I encourage you to find an accountability partner to help keep you committed

Lyons' Share Wellness | 189

to your goals throughout the process. Find a friend or co-worker who is at a similar point in his or her own journey, and agree to check in with each other daily by text message or email. Maybe this is someone who can join a gym with you, split the cost of a personal trainer, or even compare notes on meals.

Choosing an accountability partner is an important decision, so don't make the choice on a whim. Think about the type of person who will motivate you most – do you want someone to yell at you or criticize you if you slip up on a goal? Or, do you want someone who is relentlessly optimistic and will serve as your cheerleader? Do you want someone who already has made progress on his or her own health journey, or someone who is starting in the same place as you are? Do you want someone who lives nearby so you can check-in in person, or are you OK checking in by phone, email, or text message?

Before you agree to be accountability partners, agree on a check-in cadence and the length of the relationship. Are you supporting each other for a few months until you hit a goal weight, or do you intend to keep the relationship going over the long term? Ensure that both partners' expectations are set for the frequency of check-ins, so that each partner is able to support the other in the way they see fit.

If you are going to choose your significant other as an accountability partner, tread lightly. This can be enormously successful if done correctly – in fact, an Indiana University study showed that couples who worked out separately had a 43 percent dropout rate over the course of a year, versus couples who worked out together having only a 6.3 percent dropout rate over the year.[85] However, it's important to remove judgment or criticism from the process of holding your partner accountable. If one partner is able to make it to the gym more times than the other during a given week, it doesn't mean that the former partner has succeeded and the latter has failed. Make the accountability relationship about striving towards the same goal, not about comparing notes and determining a "winner."

With any accountability relationship, but especially with a significant other, it's important to focus on health, energy, and longevity – not just on how the body looks. No one wants to feel threatened that their significant other will not find them attractive if they do not go to the gym one more time or choose the salad for lunch. Choose to motivate each other at all times, rather than criticizing each other.

Choosing a Health Coach as an Accountability Partner

Of course, I think the best accountability partner of all is a Health Coach. A Health Coach is someone who is educated about health, wellness, and nutrition, but who does not prescribe one specific diet plan to his or her clients. Instead, a Health Coach helps a client improve his or her own health, by motivating the client, educating the client, and holding the client accountable. The Institute for Integrative Nutrition defines a Health Coach as "a wellness authority and supportive mentor who motivates individuals to cultivate positive health choices," and *Medical Economics* says, "The primary objectives of health coaching are to educate the patient regarding self health management and to encourage patients in taking a more proactive role in staying healthy."[86]

As a Health Coach, I hold myself responsible for providing nutrition and health information to my clients. I customize each lesson to what the particular client needs at the moment, and let the client guide the depth of information he or she receives. Some clients just want to know if eating kale or eating Twinkies is the healthier choice, while others want to know the science behind each decision. Regardless of their background, my goal is to find what will motivate and encourage the client to live his or her healthiest lifestyle. Often, this involves experimentation to figure out what is sustainable for the client's lifestyle, and what dietary and lifestyle changes work best for their unique body. It's both an art and a science, which makes it all the more rewarding when, together, we get the client feeling better than she has ever felt before.

The Value I Provide to my Clients

I often say that my health coaching programs help people "lose weight, increase their energy, or clean up their diets." However, the value of my work goes far beyond dropping the number on the scale. Most of my clients have some deeper concern when they come to me. For some, food has been the only constant getting them through an emotionally tough time, and quitting the "guilty pleasure" of binge eating is too much to bear. For others, numerous doctors have been unable to find a solution to the digestive discomforts or allergic reactions that plague them, and they are desperate for relief from their symptoms (as well as confirmation that something is, in fact, "wrong" and can be fixed).

I have worked with everyone from a 2-year-old picky eater with significant digestive issues to a 78-year-old man with numerous chronic conditions (all of which were dramatically improved with nutrition and lifestyle changes). I've worked with people who were dangerously underweight to people who had over 200 pounds to lose. I have worked with people with Type 1 and Type 2 diabetes, Hashimoto's, fibromyalgia, gout, high blood pressure, high cholesterol, cancer, chronic fatigue syndrome, eating disorders, atrial fibrillation, celiac disease, lactose intolerance, acid reflux, undiagnosed food allergies, autism, diverticulitis, epilepsy, hormonal imbalances, rheumatoid arthritis, depression, psoriasis, and many other conditions.

In all of these cases, my role as a Health Coach is not to diagnose, prescribe, or treat. Instead, my role is to educate the client on how to listen to her body, treat her body better, and respect her body enough to give it what it needs to function at its best. Whatever big goals my clients have ("lose 30 pounds," "start cooking healthy dinners for the family," or "figure out what the heck is causing me to be so bloated every night, and get rid of it!"), I break them down into bite-sized goals that the client can work on every single week. I hold the client accountable through regular check-ins to ensure that they are staying motivated and focused. By doing this, the success that I empower my clients to achieve is remarkable.

I truly do care (sometimes too much for my own good!) about my clients achieving their goals. I make it my personal mission to help them achieve what they set out to achieve, no matter what it takes. Sure, we have stumbling blocks along the way - as we experiment with different dietary strategies and motivational techniques, some are bound to work better than others. The scale never follows a perfectly linear downward path – we have to bust through plateaus, deal with celebratory weekends, and overcome other challenges. Nor is the client's overall health and well-being magically "solved" once we begin working together – the combination of stress-reduction techniques, nutrition principles, exercise routines, and more that work best for them is a complex puzzle that has to be solved over several weeks or even months. Over the long haul, though, I stand right beside my clients, encouraging them the entire way until they are happy with the outcome.

Because it would be impossible for me to summarize my clients' results in just a few pages, I've included a handful of testimonials from my current and former clients in the section titled "Testimonials" near the end of the book. Please take a moment to flip to the "Testimonials" section and browse what they say about working with me.

Recipe: How to Ensure That You Stay Motivated Daily

There are four main actions you can take after reading this chapter to ensure that you stay motivated long after you put down this book. You may choose to do just one of them, and you may eventually work your way towards all four. Remember, every journey begins with a single step, and taking the step *right now* to set up a method of keeping yourself accountable is a fantastic first step.

1. Download the *Start Here, Star There" Health Tracker* from the free bonus pack found at **www.StartHereBonus.com**. This is the tracking method I use with many of my clients, and they find great success in having daily reminders to check off these healthy behaviors.

2. Find an accountability partner to encourage you on your *Start Here* journey. You may even want to read the book together, and set goals that complement each other! Follow the guidelines listed earlier in the chapter to choose the right accountability partner for you.

3. With your accountability partner, join the Start Here Community on Facebook. Simply go to **www. StartHereCommunity.com**, and request to join. Once you do, please tag your accountability partner, and publicly state at least one health goal. Then, cheer on someone else in the group! This is an encouraging, helpful, positive, and determined group of individuals who will help you make progress towards your goals.

4. If this chapter has convinced you that a Health Coach might help you achieve your health goals, I'm happy to talk to you about the various coaching packages that I offer. Please feel free to find more information at the end of this book, visit http://www.thelyonsshare.org/health-coaching, or email me directly at megan@thelyonsshare.org.

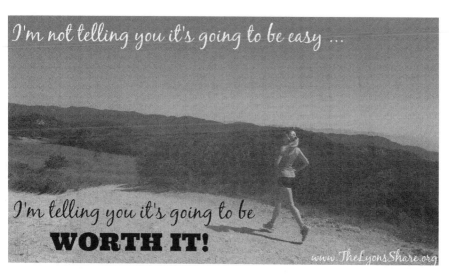

I'm not telling you it's going to be easy ...

I'm telling you it's going to be
WORTH IT!

www.TheLyonsShare.org

CHAPTER NINE

My Seven Wishes for Your Health

A Note to the Reader

*I*f you've gotten this far, thank you. Thank you from me, for reading my book, but also thank you from ... you. Thank you from the you of the future, who is more vibrant, healthy, energized, and happy because you have taken the time to prioritize your wellness. Thank you from your friends and family, who get to enjoy you for longer since you have taken some of these tips to heart. Thank you from those who you have inspired by being your healthiest and happiest self, and those you will teach by spreading some of the messages from this book.

Health doesn't have to be complicated. You don't have to follow a restrictive cleanse or participate in the latest "detox" diet. You don't have to spend hours in the kitchen every night, and you don't have to buy the fanciest, most expensive "health" products on the market. You don't have to have a "label" on your diet (think "Paleo" or "vegan" or "raw" or even "healthy"). You don't have to do what the person next to you is doing (and probably shouldn't, since your body is different from hers). You don't have to read every diet book on the market, because most of them are confusing and contradictory anyway.

Still, health is not always easy. You *do* have to get out of the warm and comfortable bed to get in your workout, even if it's just a quick 10-minute, at-home circuit workout or a brief walk outside while you're catching up with a friend. You *do* have you spend the time to plan, whether you engage in full meal preparation for the week, or just commit to using the BDD Rule and limiting your wine on your next girls' night out. You *do* have to take one small step towards your best health every single day, but you certainly, certainly, certainly don't have to be perfect.

Make a Commitment to Yourself

Throughout *Start Here*, you've gotten a variety of tips on how to improve your health. I'd like you to take a moment now to think about the areas that would benefit you most. These might not be the most comfortable things to change; in fact, you probably squirmed a little when you read these sections, getting the feeling of "I know I should do that, but I just don't really want to." Be specific, measureable, action-oriented, realistic, and time-specific (SMART) in your goals; for example, don't say, "I want to exercise more," but rather say, "I want to build up to consistently walking for 20 minutes, five times per week, by June 1st of this year." Please write your top three areas for improvement here:

1. _____

_____

_____

2. _____

_____

_____

3. _____

_____

_____

Now, go back and circle the one that you want to work on first. Make a commitment to when you will achieve this circled goal. Now, take a moment to post this goal in the Start Here Community (go to www.StartHereCommunity.com) so our encouraging group can hold you accountable.

To make this goal less overwhelming and more achievable, break it into five steps, and write them on the following lines. (For example, if you wanted to choose the walking goal I mentioned before, your steps may be: 1. Walk for 5 minutes, 3 times this week. 2. Extend the 5 minutes to 10 minutes the next week. 3. Extend the 3 times to 5 times, so I am walking 10 minutes 5 times the third week. 4. Extend the 10 minutes to 15 minutes. 5. Extend the 15 minutes to 20 minutes, so I achieve my goal in 5 weeks).

1. _____

_____

_____

2. _____

_____

_____

3. _____

_____

_____

4. _____

_____

_____

5. _____

_____

_____

This is a great start! Soon, if you stick to this plan, you will have achieved your first goal, and I hope you take the time to celebrate this achievement. Remember, it's about putting one foot in front of the other consistently, taking one small step toward the goal each day. Continuous improvement is one of the best gifts we can give ourselves. While you're on a roll, please take time to write the next 7 things you want to achieve for your health, after you achieve the first 3. You may want to practice gratitude every day, drink 80 ounces of water each day, make note of one thing you appreciate about yourself each day, experiment with meal prep, add in a veggie pack as an afternoon snack, or any number of other ideas from this book (or elsewhere). Please write them here:

1. _____

_____

_____

2. _____

_____

_____

3. _____

_____

_____

4. _____

_____

_____

5. _____

_____

_____

6. _____

_____

_____

7. _____

_____

_____

When you feel "stuck," come back to this list, and remind yourself that you have the power to improve your health!

To close the book, here are my seven wishes for your health. Please read them slowly, and take them to heart, because they certainly come straight from my own heart.

My Seven Wishes for Your Health

1. That you'll find freedom from constant worry about your diet by incorporating the seven straightforward principles outlined in this book.

2. That you'll feel vibrant, energized, and fueled to complete the activities you want to complete, whether that means playing on the floor with your great-grandchildren or conquering your first marathon.

3. That you'll find genuine appreciation and gratitude for the amazing things your body can accomplish and the wonderful life you live.

4. That you'll be strong and nourished enough to fight off chronic, life-threatening disease, as well as short-term sicknesses, fatigue, and nutrient deficiencies.

5. That you'll find a way to move your body that you truly enjoy, and that the movement will bring you stress-relief, playfulness, and fun, along with the significant health benefits.

6. That you'll find healthy foods that you love, and that you'll get joy from selecting, preparing, and eating the healthy food that nourishes your body.

7. That you'll share the gift of health with others by inspiring them to make healthy choices alongside you.

ABOUT THE AUTHOR

*M*egan Lyons wants to live in a world where healthy food has replaced the drive-thru window, where a "normal" life is a vibrant, active life, and where we rely upon our diet and lifestyle to optimize our health, rather than our medicine cabinet.

As founder and owner of The Lyons' Share Wellness, she's deeply passionate about inspiring others to feel their best. She has helped hundreds of clients lose weight, solve long-lasting digestive issues, manage chronic conditions like diabetes and high choles-

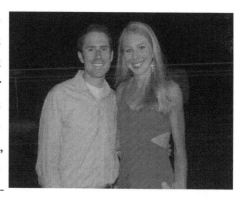

terol, learn how to feed their families healthily, and feel energized, vital, and in control of their health.

She has spoken extensively at corporations, hospitals, other medical facilities, nonprofit organizations, social groups, gyms, schools, and parent organizations.

Megan graduated with honors in economics from Harvard University in 2007, and received her MBA from Kellogg School of Management at Northwestern University in 2012. She became a Holistic Health Counselor through the Institute for Integrative Nutrition in 2011, and is currently pursuing her Masters in Holistic Nutrition from Hawthorn University.

When she's not health coaching, you can find her running, cooking, reading, traveling, and cheering on the Dallas Mavericks. She currently lives in Dallas with her husband, Kevin, and adorable dog, Maverick.

Discover how to work with Megan on the next page, or by emailing Megan@TheLyonsShare.org.

ABOUT THE LYONS' SHARE WELLNESS

*H*ave you ever struggled to maintain a healthy lifestyle, while trying to balance work, family, and a "normal" life? Have you ever gone on crash diets, only to become frustrated and return to your "old" way of living? Have you ever wanted something for your health, but found you couldn't achieve it alone?

The Lyons' Share Wellness can empower you to achieve your healthiest and happiest life.

As your Health Coach, I will listen carefully and help you to navigate the world of contradictory nutrition advice to determine what changes are necessary for you.

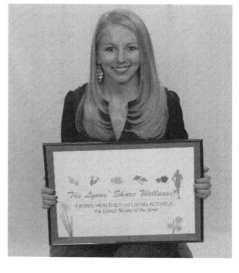

Your personalized program will radically improve your health and happiness. Together, we will explore concerns specific to you and your body and discover the tools you need for a lifetime of balance.

I currently offer four Health Coaching Programs:

- 6-month "Revolutionize"
- 3-month "Revitalize"
- 8-week "Renew"
- 8-week "Refocus"

Each Health Coaching program includes:

- Multiple one-on-one consultations (either weekly or bi-weekly, depending on your chosen program). Consultations take place by phone, Skype, or in person (in Dallas).

- Email support between sessions

- Healthy, simple-to-prepare recipes and meal planning recommendations

- Coaching and support to help you make the dietary and lifestyle changes you want

- Simple but informative handouts that will increase your nutrition knowledge

- Additional bonuses (depending on chosen program) including fitness consultations, guided grocery store tours, pantry/kitchen clean-out sessions, and more

- My personal commitment to your health and success

For information on program options, please contact **Megan@ TheLyonsShare.org.**

In addition to these Health Coaching programs, I also offer:

- Keynote presentations and workshops for audiences ranging from corporate lunch-and-learns, to patient advocate groups, to parent, social, and community organizations.

- Running coaching for all distances up to marathon, either via a personalized training plan or a personalized training plan with weekly check-ins and adjustments.

- A la carte services, such as a 50-minute "lightning round" for you to get your burning nutrition questions answered by phone, a healthy grocery shopping tour, or a pantry and kitchen clean-out.

- Food intolerance testing services, in conjunction with Alcat Laboratories.

- Corporate wellness services, including corporate presentations and "office hours" for employees.

To work with Megan, visit **www.TheLyonsShare.org/health-coaching,** or email her at Megan@TheLyonsShare.org.

TESTIMONIALS

"I've lost the weight and have been able to keep it off with a genuine smile on my face because of Megan's healthy coaching perspective and ability to tailor my eating and workout habits to my lifestyle. I contacted her while I was a grad student, who had minimal time to think about my next meal or how I was going to stick to a workout regimen, but knew that I needed to do something because I was progressively gaining weight and feeling horrible all the while. I had also been experiencing terrible digestion issues for years that I chalked off as stress-related, but Megan knew better than that.

Megan's approach of wanting to get to the bottom of my health issues with an elimination diet has changed my life. I now have so much more energy throughout the day, no longer have my embarrassing digestion issues, have been able to keep the weight off, and can still enjoy going out for food and drinks more often than I had expected. She's a great resource of information, and goes above and beyond what's expected of her because she genuinely cares. She's more than willing to find what works for you rather than forcing you do something you know you won't do. No guilt trips. Just honest, down-to-earth, professional advice. I cannot recommend her enough."

—Jennifer, grad student, Dallas

"Megan is a fountain of knowledge;, with her coaching I have lost 105 pounds eating real food and eliminating the counterproductive supplements and medications. She works by cutting through the weight- loss noise and fads. Inspiration, energy, cheerleading, recipes, and great ideas so that you no longer have the excuse not to get healthier. She finds what works for you, whether it's a paper checklist or gadgets and apps to track your health and keep you motivated."

—Steve, lawyer, Dallas

"I feel so much better after working with Megan. I'm much more aware of the food choices I'm making and the impact they have on my body. Megan is so adaptable, knowledgeable, and there's never any judgment on your choices. It's all about improving yourself and moving towards being better. It's been such a positive experience, and I'd highly recommend her to any of my friends."

—Virginia, media professional, Dallas

"Megan Lyons provides extremely useful guidance and advice for making changes in diet, nutrition, and lifestyle. As a healthcare provider, I feel confident in referring my patients to her for ongoing nutritional support and meal planning. Megan is professional, intelligent, insightful, and extremely organized! She is full of information, tips, and resources, and also a great listener. She helps me, personally, to stay focused on eating healthy, and achieving my health and wellness goals."

-Amy, acupuncturist, Dallas

"The development of the personal relationship with Megan has been the key for me.   It's been an enjoyment and it's taken something that's been a burden into something that's joyful.   The biggest benefit of health coaching with Megan is knowing that that support system is there on a daily basis if needed, by email or by phone, and knowing that Megan always has something fun for me to do. If you work with Megan, please know that this is going to be a positive experience, instead of a relentless burden, as most health programs are."

—Nancy, accountant, Dallas

"Megan was incredible. She really tried to understand my lifestyle and the challenges I face that go with it. She never advised me to just skip an event to avoid a tough situation ... rather she armed me with tips and tricks in how to be successful despite it all! Her approach to nutrition and her own passion for healthy living really served as an inspiration and motivating factor. And it worked!!!   Highly recommend her to anyone, whether you are trying to lose 50 pounds, 5 pounds or just live a healthier lifestyle."

—Tami, marketing professional, San Francisco

"After working with Megan, I have lower blood sugar levels and finally have my Type 2 diabetes under control. I've lost 13 pounds in less than 2 months. Megan has given me so much advice in terms of not just diet but lifestyle, and it's important to know that someone cares if I do well. I feel great, and I'm just thrilled with my experience."

—Brian, real estate agent, Dallas

"Working with Megan was amazing. She approaches every session with passion and commitment to getting the client exactly where he/she wants to be. Megan is interested in the whole person and attends to healthy eating, exercise, healthy cognitions and self-talk, and taking time to relax when needed (great for the busy mom!) Megan helped me focus on making the healthiest food choices for my family and even worked with my kids. She brought samples of some of her favorite grocery store healthy food choices so that I could try them out, and each session came prepared with new and exciting ideas to make meals healthy AND fun! Megan's obvious passion for health and wellness shows through and working with her was life-changing. We LOVE her!"

-Rebecca, counselor and mother, Dallas

"In addition to helping me lose and maintain 25 pounds, Megan's personalized coaching gave me the willpower to control my diet and exercise, and helped me stop feeling badly about how I felt and looked. The one-on-one contact was meaningful and important to stay focused and accountable. The most important difference is that I can honestly say I like myself more than I did before I started working with Megan."

-Pat, hospital risk manager, Baltimore

"Megan played a huge role in motivating me to stick to a healthier lifestyle. [My previous habits] made me really lethargic and fueled a vicious cycle of craving junk food when anxious/sad/stressed. Now, my boyfriend and I work out and cook together, and it's made us even closer. Plus, I've never been in better shape! Thank you!"

-Nithya, full-time graduate student, Boston

"Megan opened my eyes up to new knowledge about nutrition. I have never looked at a nutrition label the same after working with her. I know what to look for and what to avoid, and she helped me set and achieve personal goals for myself. Each week she kept me accountable to those goals and helped me with techniques on how to get my kids to eat healthier. I would recommend her to anyone looking to make changes in their – or their family's – lifestyle, no matter how healthy they are. "

-Rachel, mother, Dallas

"Megan has helped me with my diet, my 3 boys' various nutritional challenges, pregnancy nausea, and so much more. She always has plenty of meal ideas, tips and tricks, and ways to keep nutrition exciting. I highly recommend meeting with her to see how she can help you and your family!"

-Paige, mother, Dallas

"Megan helped lower my cholesterol from 220 to 160, and "rescued" me from prescription drugs. She developed a personal tracking system that taught me what worked for my body. [Her] programs also significantly improved my aches, pains, and inflammation issues. Thank you Megan – your approach, knowledge, and patience have been priceless!"

-Karen, homemaker, Dallas

"I never thought a 70-year- old man with several health complications could lose 25 pounds in 40 days ... but I did! I ate more food during the time I was working with Megan than I used to, and I feel better about my decisions. Her balance of accountability and education was perfect for me!"

–John, CPA, Dallas

"Megan was positive and easy to work with. Not only did she help keep me on track each week with my weekly goals, but she was also instrumental in helping my family eat healthier. Each week my family looked forward to trying new things for dinner and I was able to incorporate new recipes into my boring old routine. Megan exceeded my expectations and I still use her tips and tricks over a year later."

-Tiffany, mother, Dallas

"Megan is an extraordinary coach and confidante. I started working with her in the middle of a season of chaos -- - the final 6th six months before my wedding that also coincided with the start of a very demanding and time-intensive new job. While I worked with her, I ran my first half-marathon, got in incredible shape, and learned a number of things that have helped me to manage stress and maintain a healthy lifestyle while continuing to enjoy my life. She is incredibly encouraging, supportive, humble, knowledgeable, realistic, and understanding and has a special ability to break things down into achievable goals and milestones to create lasting lifestyle changes. Her passion and enthusiasm are contagious. I felt amazing, beautiful, strong, confident, and centered on my wedding day, and I owe that to Megan."

-Elise, consultant, Dallas

"Megan Lyons is top notch. As a medical professional, I've sent patients to her with confidence. All of which have thanked me for introducing Megan to them. She will sit down with you and come up with a health plan that fits your needs. She is a great resource. Her personalized, hands-on approach is just what you need. She is very knowledgeable and has numerous ways to help you live a healthier lifestyle."

-Brent, chiropractor, Dallas

"Megan not only helped me lose weight, but also helped teach our whole family healthier eating habits. She shared new recipes and encouraged new healthy habits each week. She is a kind, energetic person that I genuinely looked forward to seeing each week. After working with her, I became a happier, healthier person overall!"

-Jill, mother, Dallas

To discuss health coaching with Megan, book Megan for speaking engagements, or order books in bulk, please contact Megan@ TheLyonsShare.org.

ENDNOTES

1. International Food Information Council Foundation. Food and Health Survey, 2014. Retrieved Deecmber 12, 2014, from http://www.foodinsight.org/sites/default/files/2014 percent20Food percent20and percent20Health percent20Survey percent20Full percent20Report.pdf

2. Obesity and overweight. (2014, August 1). Retrieved December 12, 2014, from http://www.who.int/mediacentre/factsheets/fs311

3. Food Research and Action Center. Overweight and Obesity in the US. Retrieved December 12, 2014, from http://frac.org/initiatives/hunger-and-obesity/obesity-in-the-us/

4. United States Healthful Food Council, "About the United States Healthful Food Council." Retrieved February 10, 2015 from http://ushfc.org/about/#fancy-form-delay

5. Institute for Health Metrics and Evaluation. Obesity and overweight increasing worldwide. Retrieved December 12, 2014 from http://www.healthdata.org/infographic/obesity-and-overweight-increasing-worldwide

6. 2012 Food & Health Survey: Consumer Attitudes toward Food Safety, Nutrition and Health. International Food Information Council Foundation. 22 May 2012. http://www.foodinsight.org/2012_Food_Health_Survey_Consumer_Attitudes_toward_Food_Safety_Nutrition_and_Health.

7. Avena, Nicole. "The Truth Behind Fad Diets." Psychology Today. http://www.psychologytoday.com/blog/food-junkie/201307/the-truth-behind-fad-diets. July 8 2013. Accessed January 1 2015.

8. "Yo-yo Dieting Increases Type 2 Diabetes Risk." Family Practice News. http://www.familypracticenews.com/clinicaledge/obesity-weight-management/single-article/yo-yo-dieting-increases-type-2-diabetes-risk/bd3866b89c933a1044315be8c7a0f7a7.html. August 12 2014. Accessed January 1 2015.

9. International Food Information Council 2013 Food & Health Survey

10. http://www.myhealthpointe.com/health_Nutrition_news/index.cfm?Health=10 and http://miami.cbslocal.com/2013/07/02/chronic-dehydration-more-common-than-you-think/

11. Your Body's Many Cries for Water, by Fereydoon Batmanghelidj, M.D. and Integrative Nutrition, by Joshua Rosenthal

12. http://www.thedoctorstv.com/main/show_synopsis/417?section=feature&title=Boost

13. http://www.urmc.rochester.edu/encyclopedia/content. aspx?ContentTypeID=1&ContentID=1499

14. http://www.christophervasey.ch/anglais/articles/the_water_ prescription.html

15. http://www.ncbi.nlm.nih.gov/pubmed/14671205

16. http://www.thelyonsshare.org/2013/10/06/ the-health-tip-that-apples-to-75-of-americans/

17. http://www.theatlantic.com/health/archive/2013/03/ how-much-water-do-people-drink/273936/

18. http://www.ncbi.nlm.nih.gov/pubmed/19661958

19. http://www.choosemyplate.gov/food-groups/vegetables-why.html

20. http://www.ncbi.nlm.nih.gov/pubmed/23060538

21. http://www.webmd.com/food-recipes/features/ fiber-how-much-do-you-need

22. http://www.cuesa.org/learn/ how-far-does-your-food-travel-get-your-plate

23. http://www.cspinet.org/nah/articles/going-organic.html

24. http://www.ncbi.nlm.nih.gov/pubmed/20691244

25. http://www.ewg.org/foodnews/

26. Owens, Kagan, Feldman, Jay, and Kepner, John. Wide Range of Diseases Linked to Pesticides. 30(2): Summer 2010. http://www. beyondpesticides.org/assets/media/documents/health/pid-data-base.pdf.

27. Implementation of Requirements under FQPA". United States Environmental Protection Agency. September 23, 2010. http://www2. epa.gov/pesticides.

28. EWG's 2015 Dirty Dozen and Clean Fifteen. Environmental Working Group. http://www.ewg.org/foodnews/.

29. http://www.sciencedaily.com/releases/2013/05/130513174005.htm

30. http://www.usda.gov/factbook/chapter2.pdf

31. http://www.kelloggs.com/en_US/kellogg-s-cracklin-oat-bran-cereal-product.html

32. Guideline: Sugars Intake for Adults and Children. (2015). World Health Organization. Geneva, Switzerland: WHO Press. http://apps.who.int/ iris/bitstream/10665/149782/1/9789241549028_eng.pdf?ua=1

33. Ogden CL, Carroll MD, Kit BK, Flegal KM. Prevalence of childhood and adult obesity in the United States, 2011-2012. Journal of the American Medical Association 2014;311(8):806-814

34. http://www.ers.usda.gov/media/984570/sssm293.pdf

35. Basu S, Yoffe P, Hills N, Lustig RH. (2013). The Relationship of Sugar to Population-Level Diabetes Prevalence: An Econometric Analysis of Repeated Cross-Sectional Data. PLoS ONE 8(2): e57873. doi:10.1371/journal.pone.0057873.

36. Yang, Quanhe, PhD, Zhang, Zefeng, MD, Gregg, Edward W., PhD, Flanders, W. Dana, MD, ScD, Merritt, Robert, MA, and Hu, Frank B., MD, PhD. (2014). Added Sugar Intake and Cardiovascular Diseases Mortality Among US Adults. Journal of the American Medical Association Internal Medicine. 174(4): 516-524.

37. Johnson, Richard J., Segal, Mark S., Sautin, Yuri, Nakagawa, Takahiko, Feig, Daniel I., Kang, Duk-Hee, Gersch, Michael S., Benner, Steven, Sanchez-Lozada, Laura G. (2007). Potential role of sugar (fructose) in the epidemic of hypertension, obesity and the metabolic syndrome, diabetes, kidney disease, and cardiovascular disease. American Journal of Clinical Nutrition. 86:4(899-906). http://ajcn.nutrition.org/content/86/4/899.full.

38. Shanahan, Catherine, MD, and Shanahan, Luke. (2009). Deep Nutrition: Why Your Genes Need Traditional Food. Lawai, HI: Big Box Books.

39. National Research Council. Sweeteners: Issues and Uncertainties (1975). Washington, D.C.: Printing and Publishing Office, National Academy of Sciences. http://www.nap.edu/catalog/18498/sweeteners-issues-and-uncertainties.

40. Lenoir M, Serre F, Cantin L, Ahmed SH (2007) Intense Sweetness Surpasses Cocaine Reward. PLoS ONE 2(8): e698. doi:10.1371/journal.pone.0000698

41. http://www.newswise.com/articles/highly-processed-foods-dominate-u-s-grocery-purchases

42. Hidden in Plain Sight. Sugar Science: The Unsweetened Truth. http://www.sugarscience.org/hidden-in-plain-sight/#.VeYekNNViko.

43. Lenoir, M., Serre, F., Cantin, L., Ahmed, SH. Intense sweetness surpasses cocaine reward. PLoS One. 1 Aug 2007. http://www.ncbi.nlm.nih.gov/pubmed/17668074.

44. Guideline: Sugars Intake for Adults and Children. (2015). World Health Organization. Geneva, Switzerland: WHO Press. http://apps.who.int/iris/bitstream/10665/149782/1/9789241549028_eng.pdf?ua=1.

45. Howe GR, Burch JD, Miller AB, Morrison B, Gordon P, Weldon L, Chambers LW, Fodor G, Winsor GM. (1977). Artificial Sweeteners and Human Bladder Cancer. Lancet. 17:2(578-81). http://www.sciencedirect.com/science/article/pii/S0140673677914283.

46. Gallus S, Montella M, Talamini R, & Dal Maso L. (2007). Artificial sweeteners and cancer risk in a network of case-control studies. Annals of Oncology. 18(40-44). doi:10.1093/annonc/mdl346.

47. High-Intensity Sweeteners. (2014). US Food and Drug Administration. http://www.fda.gov/Food/IngredientsPackagingLabeling/FoodAdditivesIngredients/ucm397716.htm.

48. Fagherazzi G, Vilier A, Saes Sartorelli D, Lajous M, Balkau B, Clavel-Chapelon F. (2013). Consumption of artificially and sugar-sweetened beverages and incident type 2 diabetes in the Etude Epidemiologique aupres des femmes de la Mutuelle Generale de l'Education Nationale-European Prospective Investigation into Cancer and Nutrition cohort. American Journal of Clinical Nutrition. 97:3(517-523). doi: 10.3945/ajcn.112.050997.

49. Artificial Sweeteners. (2015). The Nutrition Source: Harvard School of Public Health. http://www.hsph.harvard.edu/nutritionsource/healthy-drinks/artificial-sweeteners/.

50. http://www.mayoclinic.org/healthy-lifestyle/nutrition-and-healthy-eating/in-depth/added-sugar/art-20045328

51. McGuire, Michelle, PhD, and Beerman, Kathy A., PhD. (2013). Nutritional Sciences: From Fundamentals to Food. (3). Belmont, CA: Wadsworth.

52. Salt Stats. National Center for Chronic Disease Prevention and Health Promotion. http://www.cdc.gov/Salt/pdfs/Salt_Stats_Media.pdf

53. http://edition.cnn.com/2013/05/09/sport/fauja-singh-marathon-oldest/

54. Myers, J., Kaykha, A., George, S., Abella, J., Zaheer, N., Lear, S., Yamazaki, T., Froelicher, V. Fitness versus physical activity patterns in predicting mortality in men. American Journal of Medicine 117 (12): 912-18. http://www.ncbi.nlm.nih.gov/pubmed/15629729

55. Hu, FB, Willet, WC, Li, T., Stampfer, MJ, Colditz, GA, Manson, JE. Adiposity as compared with physical activity in predicting mortality among women. New England Journal of Medicine 351(26): 2694-704. http://www.ncbi.nlm.nih.gov/pubmed/15616204/

56. Hu, FB, Willet, WC, Li, T., Stampfer, MJ, Colditz, GA, Manson, JE. Adiposity as compared with physical activity in predicting mortality among women. New England Journal of Medicine 351(26): 2694-704. http://www.ncbi.nlm.nih.gov/pubmed/15616204/

57. Blumenthal JA, Rejeski WJ, Walsh-Riddle M, Emery CF, Miller H, Roark S, Ribisl PM, Morris PB, Brubaker P, Williams RS. Comparison of high- and low-intensity exercise training early after acute myocardial infarction. Am J Cardiol. 1988 Jan 1; 61(1):26-30.

58. Helmrich, SP, Ragland, DR, Leung, RW, Paffenbarger, RS Jr. Physical activity and reduced occurrence of non-insulin-dependent diabetes mellitus. 1991. New England Journal of Medicine. 325(3): 147-52. http://www.ncbi.nlm.nih.gov/pubmed/2052059/

59. Williamson DF, Vinicor F, Bowman BA, Centers For Disease Control And Prevention Primary Prevention Working Group. Primary prevention of type 2 diabetes mellitus by lifestyle intervention: implications for health policy. Annals of Internal Medicine. 2004 Jun 1; 140(11):951-7. http://www.ncbi.nlm.nih.gov/pubmed/15172920/

60. Knowler WC, Barrett-Connor E, Fowler SE, Hamman RF, Lachin JM, Walker EA, Nathan DM, Diabetes Prevention Program Research Group. Reduction in the indicence of type 2 diabetes with lifestyle intervention or metformin. N Engl J Med. 2002 Feb 7; 346(6):393-403. http://www.ncbi.nlm.nih.gov/pubmed/11832527/

61. Hu, FB, Willet, WC, Li, T., Stampfer, MJ, Colditz, GA, Manson, JE. Adiposity as compared with physical activity in predicting mortality among women. New England Journal of Medicine 351(26): 2694-704. http://www.ncbi.nlm.nih.gov/pubmed/15616204/

62. Holmes MD, Chen WY, Feskanich D, Kroenke CH, Colditz GA. Physical activity and survival after breast cancer diagnosis. Journal of the American Medical Association. 2005 May 25; 293(20):2479-86. http://www.ncbi.nlm.nih.gov/pubmed/15914748/

63. Myers J, Kaykha A, George S, Abella J, Zaheer N, Lear S, Yamazaki T, Froelicher V. Fitness versus physical activity patterns in predicting mortality in men. American Journal of Medicine. 2004 Dec 15; 117(12):912-8. http://www.ncbi.nlm.nih.gov/pubmed/15629729/

64. The Physical Self-Perception Profile: Development and preliminary validation. Fox, Kenneth R.; Corbin, Charles B. Journal of Sport & Exercise Psychology, Vol 11(4), Dec 1989, 408-430.

65. Ranjbar, E., Memari, AH, Hafizi, S, Shayestehfar, M, Mirfazeli, FS, Eshghi, MA. Depression and Exercise: A Clinical Review and Management Guideline. Asian Journal of Sports Medicine. 2015 June; 6(2): e24055.

66. Nagamatsu LS1, Chan A, Davis JC, Beattie BL, Graf P, Voss MW, Sharma D, Liu-Ambrose T. Physical activity improves verbal and spatial memory in older adults with probable mild cognitive impairment: a 6-month randomized controlled trial. Journal of Aging Research, 2013. doi: 10.1155/2013/861893.

67. von Thiele Schwarz U, Hasson H. Employee self-rated productivity and objective organizational production levels: effects of worksite health interventions involving reduced work hours and physical exercise. Journal of Occupational Medicine. 2011 August. 53(8): 838-44. http://www.ncbi.nlm.nih.gov/pubmed/21785369.

68. Loprinzi, Paul, and Cardinal, Bradley. Association between objectively-measured physical activity and sleep. Mental Health and Physical Activity. 2011 December. 4(2):65-69. http://www.sciencedirect.com/science/article/pii/S1755296611000317.

69. Lee D, Pate RR, Lavie CJ, Sui X, Church TS, Blair SN. Leisure-Time Running Reduces All-Cause and Cardiovascular Mortality Risk. J Am Coll Cardiol. 2014;64(5):472-481. doi:10.1016/j.jacc.2014.04.058.

70. http://www.bengreenfieldfitness.com/2013/04/how-to-increase-endurance/

71. http://apps.washingtonpost.com/g/page/national/the-health-hazards-of-sitting/750/

72. https://www.washingtonpost.com/national/health-science/standing-up-at-your-desk-may-energize-you-but-it-also-may-be-tough-on-your-legs/2013/11/22/4d166d9a-0f46-11e3-8cdd-bcdc09410972_story.html

73. Patel, A., Bernstein, L., Deka, A., Feigelson, H., Campbell, P., Gapstur, S., Colditz, G., Thun, M. Leisure Time Spent Sitting in Relation to Total Mortality in a Prospective Cohort of US Adults. Am. J. Epidemiol. (2010) 172 (4): 419-429. doi: 10.1093/aje/kwq155

74. Matthews, C. E., George, S. M., Moore, S. C., Bowles, H. R., Blair, A., Park, Y., … Schatzkin, A. (2012). Amount of time spent in sedentary behaviors and cause-specific mortality in US adults. The American Journal of Clinical Nutrition, 95(2), 437–445. http://doi.org/10.3945/ajcn.111.019620

75. http://usatoday30.usatoday.com/life/lifestyle/2004-05-05-home-cooking_x.htm?csp=34

76. http://www.npr.org/blogs/thesalt/2012/11/06/164357396/restaurant-meals-means-more-calories-and-soda-for-kids-and-teens

77. http://wallblog.co.uk/2011/02/26/google-cooks-up-handy-new-recipe-view-tool/

78. http://foodpsychology.cornell.edu/outreach/large-plates.html

79. Szalavitz, Maia. "Why Gratitude isn't Just for Thanksgiving." November 12, 2012. Accessed January 2, 2015 from: http://healthland.time.com/2012/11/22/why-gratitude-isnt-just-for-thanksgiving/

80. "Gratitude and well-being: a review and theoretical integration." Clinical Psycholocy Review. November 30 2010. Accessed January 2 2015 from https://www.ncbi.nlm.nih.gov/pubmed/20451313

81. Toyota Production System. http://www.toyota.com.au/toyota/company/operations/toyota-production-system. Accessed January 1 2015.

82. http://www.forbes.com/sites/margiewarrell/2013/10/30/know-your-why-4-questions-to-tap-the-power-of-purpose/

83. Ayoko, E., Olvera, N. The Use of Social Media to Achieve Weight Loss Goals. University of Houston. https://www.coe.uh.edu/features/student-success/ayoko/eayoko_research.pdf

84. "The Power of a Gentle Nudge." Wall Street Journal. 18 May 2010. Accessed 13 March 2015. http://www.wsj.com/articles/SB10001424052 74870431490457525035240984386

85. "Strength in Numbers: The Importance of Fitness Buddies." Experience Life. July 2012. Accessed 13 March 2015. https://experiencelife.com/article/strength-in-numbers-the-importance-of-fitness-buddies/

86. "Health Coach Certification at Integrative Nutrition." http://www.integrativenutrition.com/career/healthcoaching. Accessed 15 March 2015.

Made in the USA
San Bernardino, CA
19 May 2017